Catastrophe Preparation and Prevention

for Fire Service Professionals

Principal Authors: CDR Craig Baldwin, USN (Ret.), Larry Irons, PhD, and Philip J. Palin

Principal Learning Architects: Philip J. Palin and Kari Sandhaas

The principles of prevention on which this workbook is based originated with William V. Pelfrey, PhD. The prevention cube is a tool by which these principles may be practiced. The prevention cube was conceived by Christopher Bellavita, Philip Palin, and William Pelfrey.

Teleologic Learning Company provides learning architecture for the McGraw-Hill Catastrophe Preparation series.

Higher Education

Boston   Burr Ridge, IL   Dubuque, IA   New York   San Francisco   St. Louis
Bangkok   Bogotá   Caracas   Kuala Lumpur   Lisbon   London   Madrid   Mexico City
Milan   Montreal   New Delhi   Santiago   Seoul   Singapore   Sydney   Taipei   Toronto

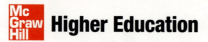

Higher Education

CATASTROPHE PREPARATION AND PREVENTION FOR FIRE SERVICE PROFESSIONALS

Published by McGraw-Hill, a business unit of The McGraw-Hill Companies, Inc., 1221 Avenue of the Americas, New York, NY 10020. Copyright © 2008 by The McGraw-Hill Companies, Inc. All rights reserved. No part of this publication may be reproduced or distributed in any form or by any means, or stored in a database or retrieval system, without the prior written consent of The McGraw-Hill Companies, Inc., including, but not limited to, in any network or other electronic storage or transmission, or broadcast for distance learning.

Some ancillaries, including electronic and print components, may not be available to customers outside the United States.

This book is printed on acid-free paper.

1 2 3 4 5 6 7 8 9 0 DOW/DOW 0 9 8 7

ISBN 978-0-07-338285-2
MHID 0-07-338285-X

Vice President/Editor in Chief: *Elizabeth Haefele*
Vice President/Director of Marketing: *John E. Biernat*
Publisher: *Linda Schreiber*
Managing Developmental Editor: *Sarah Wood*
Marketing Manager: *Kelly Curran*
Lead Media Producer: *Damian Moshak*
Media Producer: *Marc Mattson*
Director, Editing/Design/Production: *Jess Ann Kosic*
Senior Project Manager: *Rick Hecker*
Production Supervisor: *Janean A. Utley*
Designer: *Srdj Savanovic*
Media Project Manager: *Mark A. S. Dierker*
Cover/Interior/CD Designer & Illustrator: *Kari Sandhaas, Teleologic Learning Company*
Typeface: *10/13.5 Frutiger Light*
Printer: *R R Donnelley, Willard, OH*

San Luis Rey® is a registered service mark of Teleologic Learning (LLC).
The credit section for this book begins on page 153 and is considered an extension of the copyright page.

Library of Congress Control Number: 2007934406

www.mhhe.com

"A **CATASTROPHE** IS ANY NATURAL OR MANMADE INCIDENT, including terrorism, that results in extraordinary levels of mass casualties, damage or destruction severely affecting the population, infrastructure, environment, economy, national morale, and/or government functions. A catastrophic event could result in sustained national impacts over a prolonged period of time; almost immediately exceeds resources normally available to state, local, tribal, and private-sector authorities in the impacted area; and significantly interrupts governmental operations and emergency services to such an event that national security could be threatened."

— THE NATIONAL RESPONSE PLAN

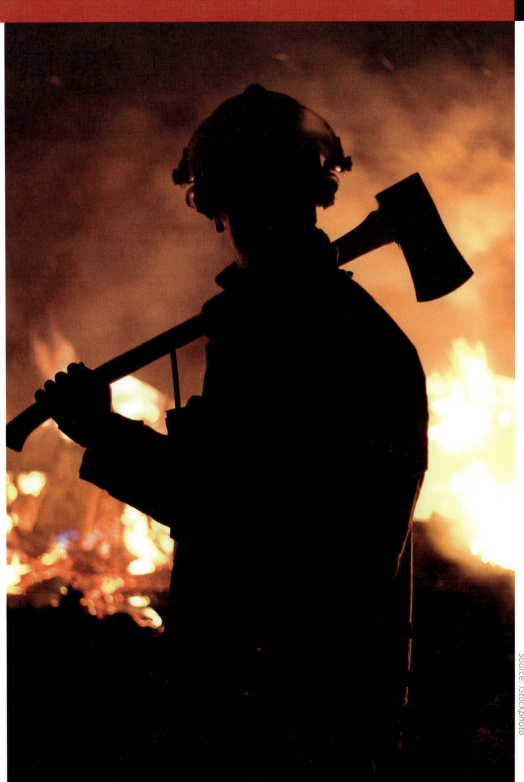

Source: iStockphoto

Catastrophe Preparation and Prevention for Fire Service Professionals
is the second in a series of titles available from The McGraw-Hill Companies. Other titles include:

Catastrophe Preparation and Prevention for Law Enforcement Professionals (previously published)
Catastrophe Preparation, Prevention and Response for Law Enforcement Professionals
Catastrophe Preparation, Prevention, Response, and Recovery for Law Enforcement Professionals

Catastrophe Preparation, Prevention and Response for Fire Service Professionals
Catastrophe Preparation, Prevention, Response, and Recovery for Fire Service Professionals

Catastrophe Preparation and Prevention for Emergency Medical Services Professionals
Catastrophe Preparation, Prevention and Response for Emergency Medical Services Professionals
Catastrophe Preparation, Prevention, Response, and Recovery for Emergency Medical Services Professionals

Catastrophe Preparation and Prevention for Public Health Professionals
Catastrophe Preparation, Prevention and Response for Public Health Professionals
Catastrophe Preparation, Prevention, Response, and Recovery for Public Health Professionals

Catastrophe Preparation and Prevention for Public Services Professionals
Catastrophe Preparation, Prevention and Response for Public Services Professionals
Catastrophe Preparation, Prevention, Response, and Recovery for Public Services Professionals

Catastrophe Preparation and Prevention for Elected Officials
Catastrophe Preparation, Prevention and Response for Elected Officials
Catastrophe Preparation, Prevention, Response, and Recovery for Elected Officials

Catastrophe Preparation: Key Issues in Inter-Agency Collaboration

Catastrophe Preparation: Key Issues in Civil-Military Collaboration

Catastrophe Preparation: Key Issues in Regional Collaboration

Catastrophe Preparation: Key Issues in Intergovernmental Collaboration

TABLE OF CONTENTS

iv	ORIENTATION

1   CHAPTER 1 — Introduction
- Prevention Basics
- Aligning Local and National Strategy
- Catastrophe, Risk Management, and Real Life
- Natural, Accidental, and Intentional Threats
- Practicing Prevention
- Intentional Threats: Challenging our Imagination
- Chapter Review
- Apply What You Have Learned

25   CHAPTER 2 — Recognize Threats
- Who and/or What
- Your Local History
- Weapons of Catastrophe
- Vulnerability
- Consequences
- Fear as a Threat Amplifier
- Chapter Review
- Apply What You Have Learned

51   CHAPTER 3 — Share Information
- Strategic Intelligence and Fire Intelligence
- The Intelligence Process
- Choose Intelligence Targets
- Collecting Data and Information
- Organize and Analyze Data and Information
- Produce Intelligence Products
- Consume Intelligence Products
- Chapter Review
- Apply What You Have Learned

84   CHAPTER 4 — Collaborate
- Defining Collaboration
- Collaboration Process
- Designing a Collaborative Network
- Collaboration and Sharing Information
- Collaboration and Identifying Targets
- Regional Collaboration
- Collaborative Agreements
- Chapter Review
- Apply What You Have Learned

110   CHAPTER 5 — Manage Risk
- Current Priorities
- Apply a Risk Formula
- SARA and RISK Management
- Choosing Among Risks
- Scenario-Based Risk Assessment
- A Collaborative Choice
- TARA: Four Responses to Risk
- Continually Assess Your Choice
- Chapter Review
- Apply What You Have Learned

131   CHAPTER 6 — Decide to Intervene
- The Prevention Cube: What and When?
- Primary Mode: Protect, Deter, and Preempt
- Secondary Mode: Protect, Deter, and Preempt
- Tertiary Mode: Protect, Deter, and Preempt
- Making an Effective Decision
- Planning and Resourcing
- Preparing for Catastrophe
- Chapter Review
- Apply What You Have Learned

153	ACKNOWLEDGMENTS
155	WORKS CITED
161	APPENDIX — San Luis Rey
170	GENERAL INDEX

ORIENTATION — LEARNING MAP

Where does this workbook take you?

PREVENTION CUBE

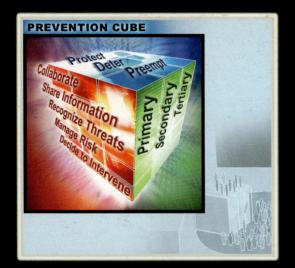

END HERE
Achieve your goal to **prevent or mitigate** catastrophe in your community.

Have you reached your goal by applying a principled process?

DECIDE TO INTERVENE — 6
You must **plan, resource, train, exercise, and triage** so you are ready to intervene.

Can you effectively intervene?

BEGIN HERE — 1
Your goal is to prevent or mitigate catastrophe.

Use a **principled process** to move forward, but know that uncertainties and obstacles lie ahead.

Will you be able to successfully negotiate them?

Chapter 1

Chapter 6

Chapter 2

RECOGNIZE THREATS — 2
Threats can be **natural**, **accidental**, or **intentional**.

Will you recognize who or what your threats are?

| RECOGNIZE THREATS | SHARE INFORMATION | COLLABORATE |

ORIENTATION — LEARNING MAP v

MANAGE RISK 5

Risk = Likelihood x Consequences

Likelihood = Threat { x **Vulnerability** *if (state conditions)*
/ **Vulnerability** *if (state conditions)*

Choose wisely.
Transfer, **A**void, **R**educe, or **A**ccept Risk.
Can you accurately identify your risks?

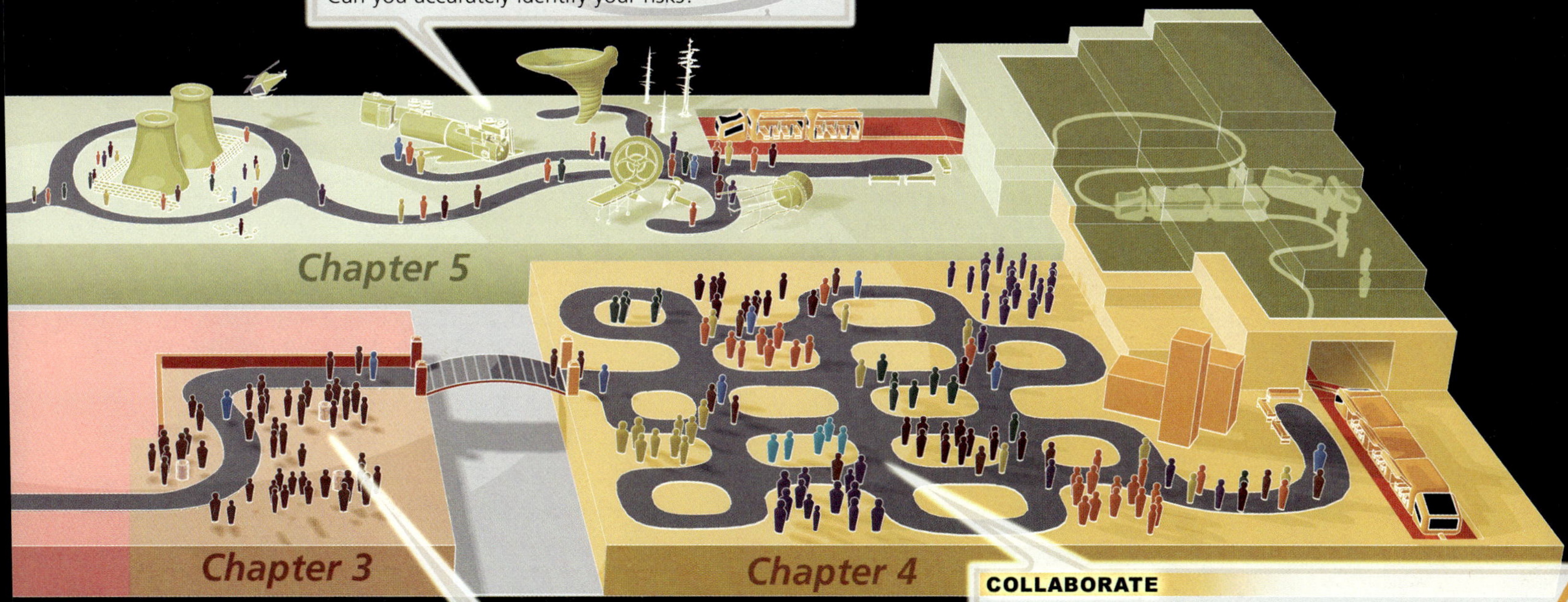

Chapter 5

Chapter 3

Chapter 4

SHARE INFORMATION 3

You must understand **threat capabilities**, know your **vulnerabilities**, and envision **consequences**.

Obstacles abound. Can you overcome them?

COLLABORATE 4

To succeed you must form **strategic partnerships**, craft **effective networks**, and generate **mutual self interest**.

There are many different paths to collaboration.

Which will lead you to where you need to go?

MANAGE RISK | DECIDE TO INTERVENE

You don't understand anything until you learn it more than one way.

—MARVIN MINSKY
Professor Emeritus, MIT

WORKBOOK COMPONENTS

There are six chapters in this workbook. The first provides an introduction to concepts and fundamentals detailed in subsequent chapters. Chapters two through six offer explanations, examples, and suggestions for implementing effective ways to prevent or reduce the risk of catastrophe in your community.

Each chapter begins with a list of **learning objectives**. Each chapter ends with a set of **review questions** that you should be able to answer by the time you reach that point in the workbook. If you cannot answer a question, a second reading of what you missed is a wise idea.

APPLIED LEARNING

Throughout the workbook you will be asked **questions specifically related to your own community**. These questions are flagged by a blue **community icon**. You already know the answers to most of these questions. The biggest benefit you derive from this workbook may be the experience of describing and organizing what you already know—thus, enabling you to apply those understandings more effectively in your community. Take the time to write out your answers in the spaces provided. This is a good way to practice applying essential concepts and to collect notes for making your case on the job.

"San Luis Rey®"

Further opportunities for applied learning are offered through instructional activities utilizing the **fictional jurisdiction of San Luis Rey®**. San Luis Rey is a composite based on real-world places and problems. It was developed to provide a rich environment for exploring prevention and preparedness problems you are likely to encounter in the real world. Testing concepts and honing decision-making skills within a fictional environment offers a risk-free training ground for developing life-preserving skills and understanding.

San Luis Rey® is a registered service mark of Teleologic Learning LLC (www.teleologic.net).

ORIENTATION

Online Exercises

Following each chapter review is an invitation to reinforce your learning through enrollment and participation in a game-like **online exercise** offered by the Institute for Preventive Strategies. These exercises are focused on preventing a terrorist attack within the fictional environment of San Luis Rey. Access instructions and a brief segue to the appropriate exercise are located in the **Apply What You Have Learned** section at the end of each workbook chapter.

Open Source Daily Brief

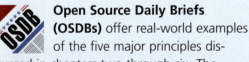 **Open Source Daily Briefs (OSDBs)** offer real-world examples of the five major principles discussed in chapters two through six. The Institute for Preventive Strategies distributes online OSDBs every weekday morning. When you sign up for the online exercise you will begin to receive these action briefings.

FOUNDATIONAL PRINCIPLES

The Prevention Cube

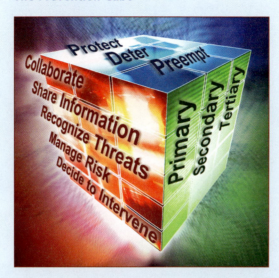

Both the online exercise and this workbook are based on a problem-solving framework called the "**prevention cube**." When you have completed this workbook you will understand how to use the principles of the prevention cube to prevent or reduce the risk of catastrophe in your community.

ILLUSTRATION ON NEXT PAGE: *1938 fire in downtown Bloomington, IL. Inset postcard: 1901 fire, Peoria, IL. Source: Historic photos courtesy of the Bloomington Fire Department, Bloomington, IL*

Excerpt by Benjamin Franklin, "Protection of Towns from Fire," February 4, 1735 issue of The Pennsylvania Gazette, written under the alias, "old citizen."

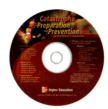

Using the CD

In a sleeve inside the back cover is a Compact Disc. This CD is packed with information you can use to deepen your familiarity with the main topics introduced in the workbook. The **resources** on the CD are more than five times the size of the workbook—including books, articles, and links to online sources. Many of these resources are referenced throughout the workbook and listed in the Works Cited section at the back.

Throughout the workbook you will see this **CD icon:** 💿 This symbol identifies a relevant resource that is available on the CD. It is especially convenient to use the workbook at the same time as you also have the CD content open in your computer's browser. This way you can check to see if the additional background is relevant to your needs or interests.

The CD also provides access to an online exercise in preventing a terrorist attack. This highly interactive, game-like exercise will help you apply the workbook lessons. At the end of each chapter you are encouraged to access a specific part of the exercise that deals with the focus of that particular chapter.

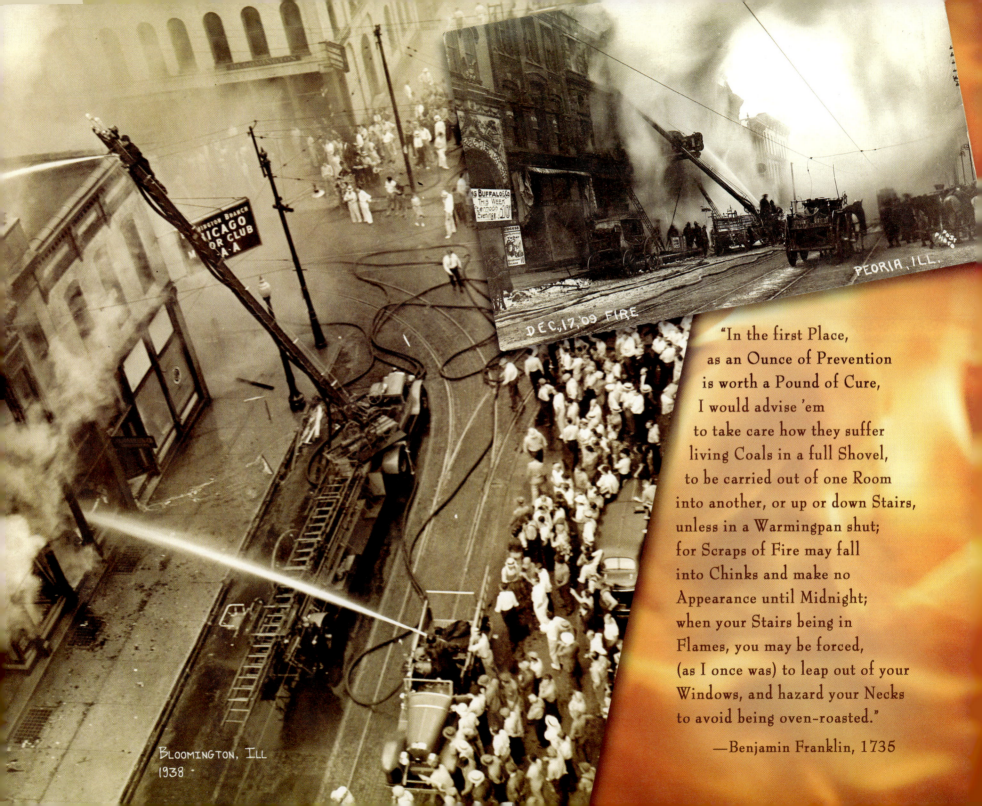

BLOOMINGTON, ILL 1938

DEC. 17, '09 FIRE — PEORIA, ILL.

"In the first Place, as an Ounce of Prevention is worth a Pound of Cure, I would advise 'em to take care how they suffer living Coals in a full Shovel, to be carried out of one Room into another, or up or down Stairs, unless in a Warmingpan shut; for Scraps of Fire may fall into Chinks and make no Appearance until Midnight; when your Stairs being in Flames, you may be forced, (as I once was) to leap out of your Windows, and hazard your Necks to avoid being oven-roasted."

—Benjamin Franklin, 1735

CHAPTER 1 — INTRODUCTION

Introduction

✓ *In this chapter you will learn:*

- How you already manage risk.
- How to categorize threats.
- How to differentiate between a disaster and a catastrophe.
- How to give special attention to prevention.
- How to recognize the special characteristics of intentional threats.

WHENEVER THE COMMUNITY IS THREATENED—FROM WHEREVER BY WHATEVER—FIRE SERVICE PROFESSIONALS WANT TO BE THERE TO DEFEND THEIR NEIGHBORS.

In the aftermath of disaster, the fire service is there to care for the victims, protect property, and defend the powerless. In advance of a disaster, the fire service plans, trains, and exercises with other preparedness professionals to stand ready for the disaster.

Prevention, as Benjamin Franklin noted, is a key part of fire safety. In 1736, Franklin founded the Union Fire Company in Philadelphia. This became the model for volunteer fire company organization (Hashagen, "Firefighting in Colonial America"). Volunteer firefighters continue as a crucial part of the fire service.

Prevention principles have long been a key component of firefighter training and practice. These principles include collaboration through public education, training with other public safety agencies, "gathering intelligence" through fire inspections and fire investigations, recognizing threats through systematic analysis of service calls and fire events, and managing risk through fire codes, building codes, and zoning regulations.

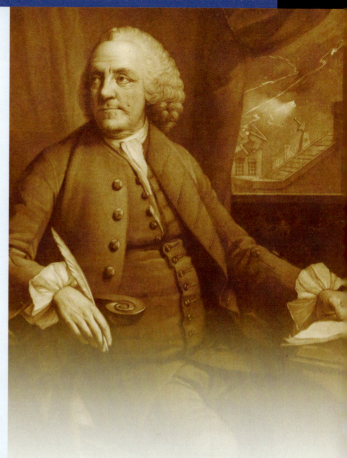

An Ounce
of Prevention
is worth
a Pound of Cure…

—Benjamin Franklin

ABOVE: *Benjamin Franklin. Source: Library of Congress*

CHAPTER 1 — INTRODUCTION

PREVENTION BASICS

The fire service is already engaged in a range of activities that are—or can be—crucial to effective prevention of natural, accidental, and intentional catastrophes.

Fire chiefs, police chiefs, and line-level professionals in many preparedness professions indicate the public finds the fire service easier to approach than law enforcement. Members of the fire service regularly enter more homes, offices, factories, and warehouses than do other first responders. The fire prevention work of many departments results in a strong network of community relationships through schools, civic organizations, and places of worship. The public's trust in the fire service—and its wide-ranging activities—allows the fire service to be a community's eyes-and-ears.

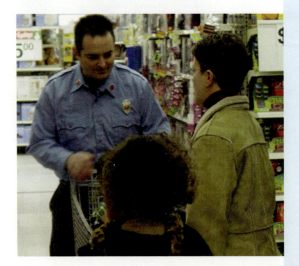

The public considers the men and women of the fire service among the easiest first responder professions to approach.

This approachability can contribute to the role of fire service in terrorism prevention.

Gathering information about communities and the hazards they face is a central practice of fire service professionals in their response and preventive work (Mitchell, Doherty, and Hibbard). Fire service professionals need critical building information, such as floor plans and plot plans of an area. The Los Angeles Fire Department's Building Inventory Program gathers information from "pre-fire" inspections, standardizes it, and places a copy on every fire apparatus in the city. The information is useful to firefighters responding to incidents in previously assessed properties. Access to and familiarity with this information gives the fire service a unique role to play in assessing the strengths and vulnerabilities of our communities.

Fire service professionals already support crime prevention by minimizing building dilapidation and abandonment through enforcement of local building codes, thereby limiting a basic environmental factor in street crime. In several communities the fire service plans and works with other public safety professions in a joint effort to enhance the overall safety of targeted areas. In many communities the fire service is unique in proactive engagement with the private sector, extending to joint inspections and shared training. The experience of the fire service in working collaboratively with other governmental agencies and the private sector is an important foundation for addressing catastrophic threats.

CHAPTER 1 — INTRODUCTION

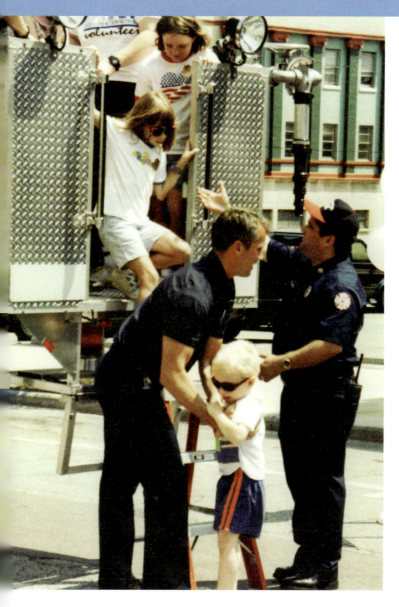

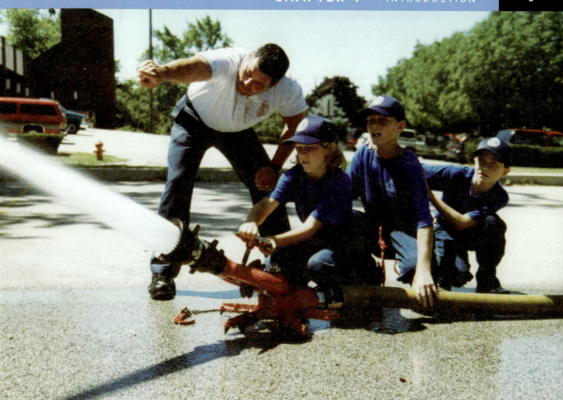

Many Fire Departments conduct outreach and public education programs resulting in increased cooperation and trust from their community.

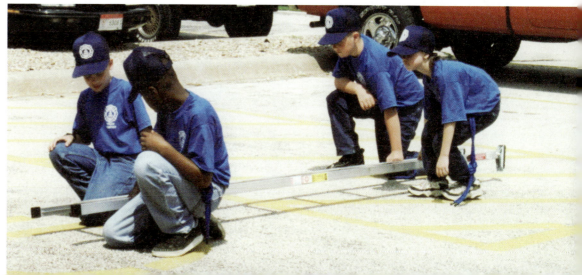

ABOVE and RIGHT: *Bloomington firefighters conducting community educational programs. Bloomington, IL*

PREVIOUS PAGE: *Bloomington Fire Department collaborates with Bloomington Police Department in a holiday "Shop with a Cop and Firefighter" program. (Upper: Eric Vaughn; Lower: Joe Hoeniges)*

Photos courtesy of the Bloomington Fire Department, Bloomington, IL

CHAPTER 1 — INTRODUCTION

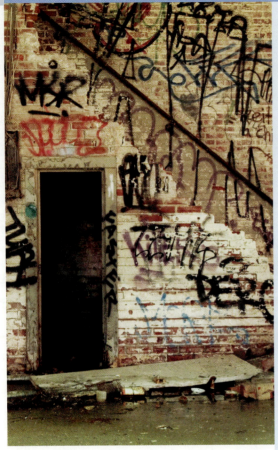

Source: iStockphoto

Fire service professionals minimize building dilapidation and abandonment through enforcement of local building codes.

This, in turn, helps prevent street crime by eliminating environments that may harbor criminal activity.

ALIGNING LOCAL AND NATIONAL STRATEGY

Most local fire departments would readily agree they have a role to play in preventing accidental disasters. Many would recognize a role in reducing the risk of natural calamities. But when it comes to intentional—terrorist—threats many fire departments underestimate their potential role in prevention.

The **top three strategic objectives of the National Strategy for Homeland Security**, in order of priority, are:

1. **preventing terrorist attacks within the United States**
2. **reducing America's vulnerability to terrorism**
3. **minimizing the damage and recovering from attacks that may occur**

Recent studies of counterterrorism initiatives by the fire departments of Los Angeles and New York City have found the fire service can play an important role. According to those involved in the studies, educating fire service professionals about how to recognize the roles and motivations of individual terrorists, their cell systems, fundraising, and the street-level mechanics of terrorist operations is the best way for the fire service to contribute to terrorism prevention (Welch; Flynn, John). Along with law enforcement, emergency management, public health, public works, and others the fire service is a crucial participant in all three strategic objectives.

Fire departments across the nation are experienced in working with other public safety agencies in responding to incidents. This response capability has been enhanced in recent years through implementation of the National Incident Management System (NIMS). The explicit goal of NIMS is to establish a collaborative framework for inter-governmental (federal, state, tribal, territorial, and local), inter-agency (such as law, fire, and public heath) and public-private (including critical infrastructure owners and operators) cooperation in incident management.

Prevention is aimed at avoiding the incident in the first place. Prevention of catastrophe—natural, accidental, or intentional—is the first objective of the National Strategy. Helping the fire service play a leading role in prevention is the goal of this workbook. As such, much of the following is outside the scope of NIMS as currently conceived.

Using tools of protection, deterrence, and preemption, fire service professionals can contribute to the prevention of catastrophe. Inspections done to prevent damage from fire, flood, earthquake, or wind also provide opportunities to observe unusual patterns, notice atypical chemical odors, or recognize unnecessary and dangerous risks to critical infrastructure. Radiation detectors carried by many fire departments provide the means to detect radiation in unusual locations. All of these opportunities—and more—are potential sources of information on terrorist activity or accident-conducive conditions.

A disaster often becomes a catastrophe when a threat interacts in an unexpected way with existing infrastructure. In the case of the September 11 attacks, even Osama bin Laden was surprised by the collapse of the World Trade Center towers. It can be argued it was not Hurricane Katrina that brought catastrophe to New Orleans; rather it was the failure of a few key levees.

By both tradition and mission the fire service has particular expertise regarding the infrastructure of the community. Because of what you already know and do, fire service professionals can play a critical role in preventing catastrophe. In many ways it is a specialized intelligence role:

- Recognizing and reducing risks to infrastructure in advance of any incident;

- Sharing knowledge regarding locally available hazardous materials that can seriously amplify a natural, accidental, or intentional threat; and

- Using your broadly based and widely trusted eyes-and-ears as a community early warning system for unusual patterns or behavior that could suggest increased risk.

This specialist intelligence role does not require a fundamental shift in what most Fire Departments already understand as their primary mission. But it may involve a new awareness of how your expertise can be helpful to other preparedness professions.

The terrorist threat has global roots. Yet, its thorny flowers blossom in someone's hometown: Oklahoma City, New York City, London, Beslan, Glasgow and dozens more towns large and small. Today's terrorists are largely decentralized and depend on their local knowledge and networks. Terrorists seek to attack in unexpected ways. Terrorists use their local know-how to amplify the impact of their attacks.

The fire service has unique local knowledge and premier local networks to contribute to preventing terrorism and reducing each community's risk of natural, accidental, or intentional catastrophe.

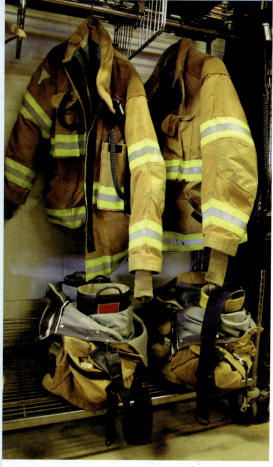

Source: iStockphoto

Every citizen should be attentive to the risks facing their community.

Fire service professionals bring to this task specific skills and strengths. They are on the front-line and at the bottom-line of each community's ability to prevent, respond, and recover.

CHAPTER 1 — INTRODUCTION

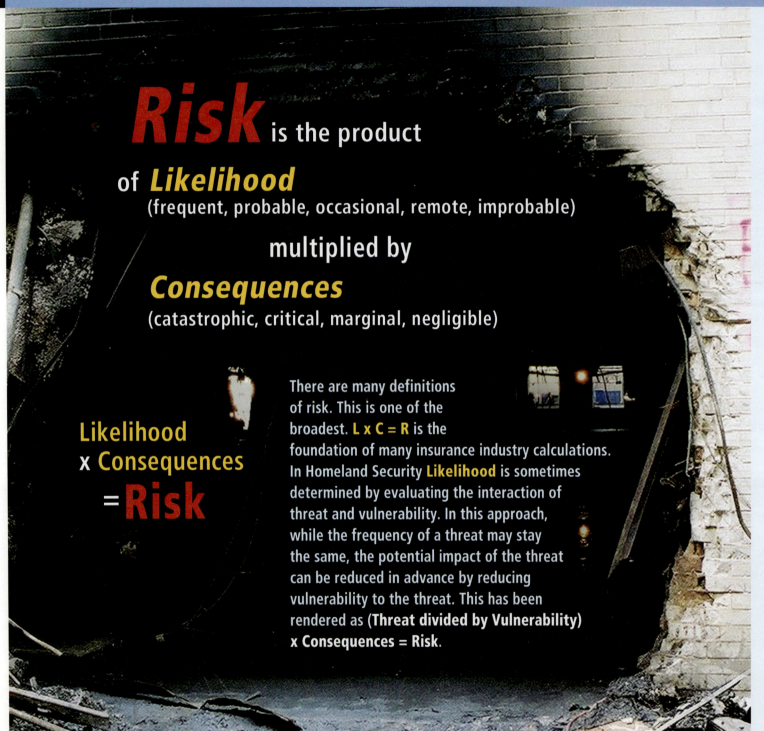

Risk is the product

of **Likelihood**
(frequent, probable, occasional, remote, improbable)

multiplied by

Consequences
(catastrophic, critical, marginal, negligible)

**Likelihood
x Consequences
= Risk**

There are many definitions of risk. This is one of the broadest. **L x C = R** is the foundation of many insurance industry calculations. In Homeland Security **Likelihood** is sometimes determined by evaluating the interaction of threat and vulnerability. In this approach, while the frequency of a threat may stay the same, the potential impact of the threat can be reduced in advance by reducing vulnerability to the threat. This has been rendered as **(Threat divided by Vulnerability) x Consequences = Risk**.

LEFT:
Hole in the Pentagon wall, after September 11, 2001 terrorist attack.

CHAPTER 1 — INTRODUCTION

CATASTROPHE, RISK MANAGEMENT, AND REAL LIFE

Risk is inherent to firefighting. Every rookie learns the fundamentals of managing their risks—or they may not make it past being a rookie. The most seasoned firefighter knows there are plenty of risks that persist. Making a choice—often a split second choice—between which risk to take and which to avoid can mean the difference between life and death, yours and others'.

The same kind of choice is key to preparing for catastrophes. The world is full of risks: terrorists, accidental explosions, tornadoes, earthquakes, pandemics (intentional, accidental, or natural), and much more. Fire service professionals need to prepare for all these risks. **But preparing for catastrophe is very different from preparing for everyday risks.**

A big part of the difference is psychological. **The more likely and near-term the perceived risk, the more attention we give it. The less likely and less immediate the risk the more we are tempted to discount it.** This is not always a bad choice. However, when taken to an extreme—if we basically ignore the less likely but catastrophic threats—we put our communities and ourselves at extreme risk.

There is clear evidence of catastrophic risk. Terrorist attacks, killer hurricanes, earthquakes, floods, hazardous material spills, "dirty" bombs, chemical explosions, building fires, wildfires, and potential pandemics are regular features on the nightly news. There is a clear need for the fire service and other preparedness professionals to develop a shared means of thinking about, planning, and working together to manage the risk of catastrophic events.

Certainly this thinking, planning, and working includes being able to respond effectively to a catastrophe.

With catastrophic risks, being prepared to respond is not enough. We want to prevent catastrophes. When we cannot prevent, we at least want to reduce the impact of the catastrophe. In every case we want to be prepared to recover from the catastrophe as quickly and effectively as possible.

While the challenge is different we **manage these extraordinary risks with the same basic tools with which we manage our more ordinary risks:** we recognize them, analyze them, plan for them, train for them, and prepare our minds, skills, and organizations to deal with them.

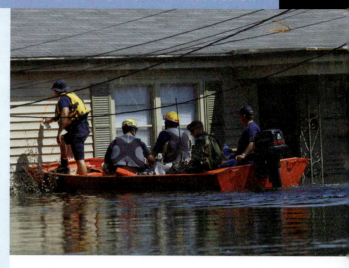

ABOVE: *Rescue personnel from the Los Angeles Fire Department, the U.S. Coast Guard (USCG), and the U.S. Army (USA) search for survivors of Hurricane Katrina in a flooded New Orleans neighborhood, September 11, 2005*
Source: *U.S. Dept. of Defense photo by PH1(AW/SW) Robert McRill, USN*

NEXT PAGE:
Aftermath of Hurricane Katrina in New Orleans, 2005.
Source: *Fifth U.S. Army/U.S. Army North*

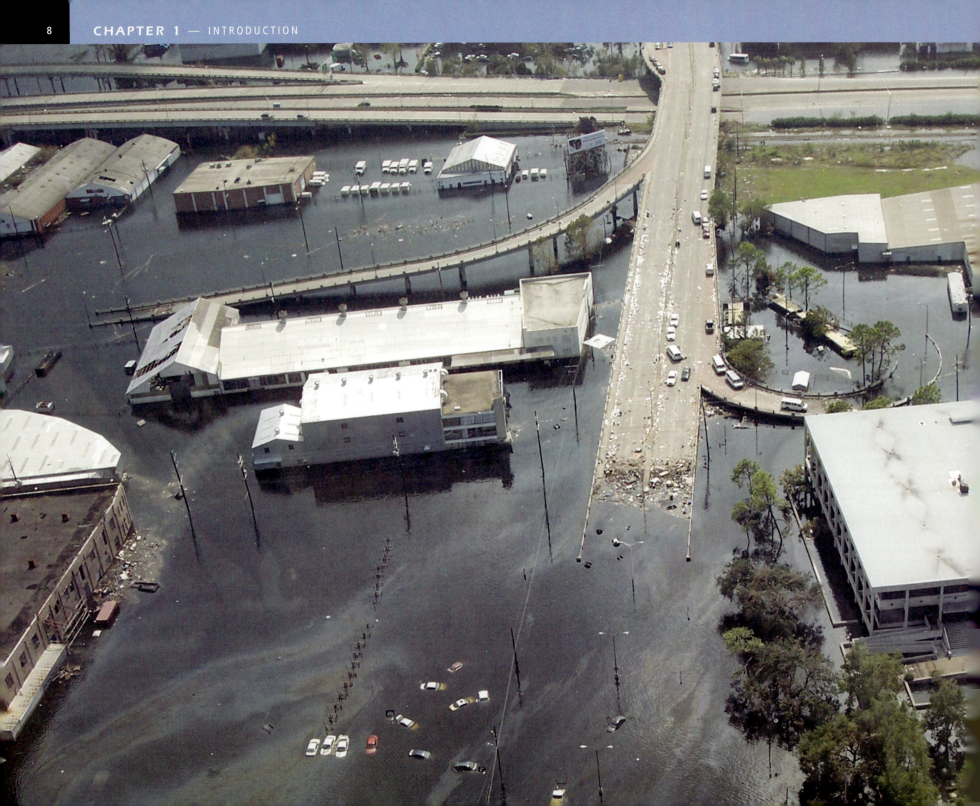

CHAPTER 1 — INTRODUCTION

NATURAL, ACCIDENTAL, AND INTENTIONAL THREATS

Fire service personnel are accustomed to dealing with a wide range of threats: motor vehicle, residential, industrial, or high-rise fires, hazardous material spills, radiological exposure, and more.

Catastrophes come in three basic types:

Natural catastrophes generally have their origins in weather events or geological events, or the interaction of the two. Examples include hurricanes, tornadoes, flooding, volcanic eruptions, earthquakes, tsunamis, heat emergencies, drought, and wild fires. Biological catastrophes such as the Black Death and the 1918 Spanish Flu Pandemic are less common but have much broader impacts. While we cannot usually prevent natural catastrophes, actions taken in advance to reduce vulnerability can lessen the damage along with effective response and recovery operations.

Accidental catastrophes are the result of unintentional human error or negligence. Accidents may also compound the impact of natural and intentional catastrophes. Examples include procedural errors in chemical or nuclear operations, dam failures, truck collisions involving toxic materials, train derailments or collisions involving toxic materials, design or engineering failures involving large structures, controlled burns escaping containment, and decisions or non-decisions that increase the vulnerability of large populations in response to an emergency. Accidental catastrophes are, in principle, preventable through enhanced planning, training, and exercising. Given human nature, it is probably more accurate to say we can reduce the likelihood and impact of accidental catastrophes.

Intentional catastrophes are the result of purposeful human decisions to cause death and destruction. Examples include terrorism, warfare, and genocide. Since the emergence of modern medicine, human intention has killed more people than natural and accidental catastrophes combined. Given their origins in human purpose, intentional catastrophes are the most preventable. We can identify people with a deadly purpose and prevent them from acting. Over time, benign purposes sometimes replace aggressive ones. After many centuries of hostility, Germany and France still compete, but war between them—at least today—seems very unlikely.

Though accidental and intentional catastrophes are both man-made, in the sense that human activity causes both, distinguishing between the two in discussing prevention is important. Intentional threats typically involve deception and deadly purpose. Accidents typically involve harm to people and property resulting from unintentional consequences stemming from non-lethal purposes.

Intentional catastrophes are the most

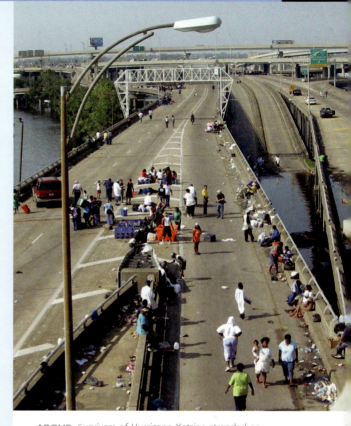

ABOVE: *Survivors of Hurricane Katrina stranded on Highway 10 in New Orleans. September 1, 2005 Source: DefenseLink photo by CMSGT Gonda Moncada, USAF*

Were the worst impacts of Hurricane Katrina on New Orleans the result of natural or accidental causes?

Have you, your family, or your community ever experienced a catastrophe? (circle one)

yes   no

How did the catastrophe differ from other difficult—or even disastrous—events?

_____
_____
_____
_____
_____
_____
_____
_____
_____
_____

Mitigation means to soften the results of harm.

The harm happens but it is less intense or less serious than the results when preventive steps go untaken in advance to mitigate the harm.

susceptible to prevention, but given human creativity are especially difficult to predict.

Death and destruction are common. Firefighters know this better than most. But, **a catastrophe is a disaster with a scope and scale that implies an effective response is very difficult and full recovery impossible.**

A catastrophe is an event so disastrous that it changes everything for always. The ancient Greek term from which the word derives means "an irreversible change in direction." According to Federal Judge Richard Posner a catastrophe is, "an event that is believed to have a very low probability of materializing but that if it does materialize will produce a harm so great and sudden as to seem discontinuous with the flow of events that preceded it." (*Catastrophe: Risk and Response*)

To the extent that the current flow of events—our civic life, our family situation, our economic prospects, our place in the world—is satisfactory to us, then we want to prevent catastrophes. The risk of an entirely new—and largely unpredictable—flow of events is something we want to avoid.

There are, however, thousands of individuals who do not consider a fundamental shift in the flow of events a significant risk. They are so dissatisfied with the current course of their lives that they consider a great and sudden change—almost any sort of change—an improvement in their prospects.

To the satisfied, catastrophe is a threat. To the dissatisfied, catastrophe is an opportunity. As a result, intentional catastrophe has become a particularly dangerous threat.

But catastrophe—natural, accidental, or intentional—is not on the mind of most citizens or fire service personnel. Both San Francisco and St. Louis sit on or near major earthquake faults. A catastrophe is likely. New Orleans was clearly unprepared for a long-predicted catastrophe. Many studies and experts predict that terrorists will utilize biological or nuclear weapons that threaten tens of thousands of deaths. Are we giving any more attention to these warnings than we did to the probability of a Category 3 or worse hurricane in Lake Pontchartrain?

Attention to low-probability but high-impact threats requires a discipline and professionalism that is unusual.

One of the hard-won benefits of the 9/11 attacks, Hurricane Katrina, and the prospect of a new pandemic is recognition that protecting the community now requires attention to catastrophic threats, and especially to the prevention and mitigation of catastrophe.

Once a true catastrophe occurs, the options are very limited. Looking ahead and working ahead to prevent and mitigate catastrophe is the only effective option.

CHAPTER 1 — INTRODUCTION

CATASTROPHE
an event so disastrous that it
changes everything for always

We certainly must be prepared to *respond* to catastrophe.

But we never really *recover* from a true catastrophe.

CHAPTER 1 — INTRODUCTION

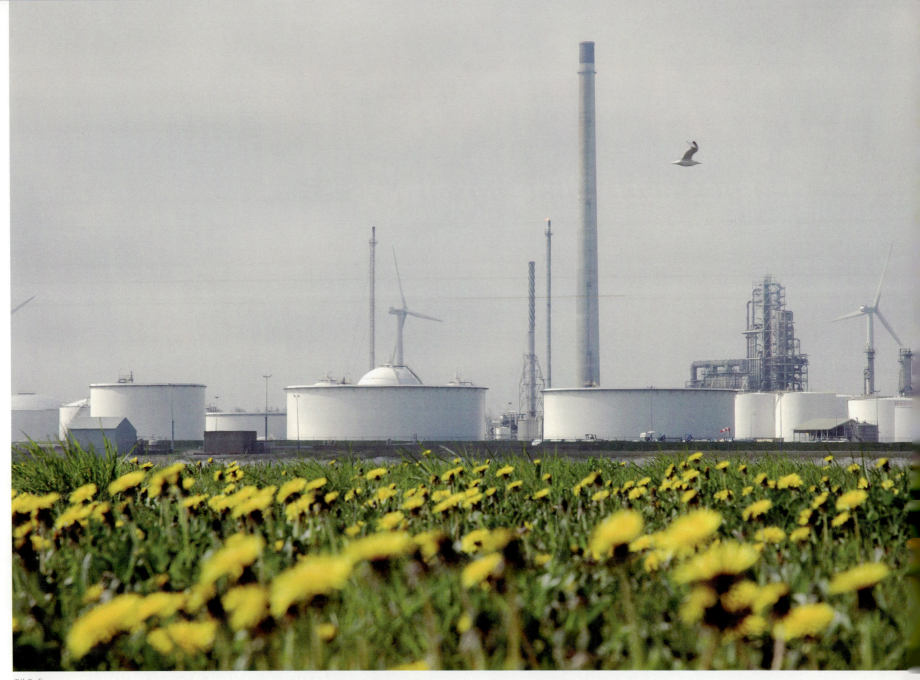

Oil Refinery
Source: iStockphoto

Terrorists make strategic choices based on what they see as vulnerabilities.

PRACTICING PREVENTION

Collaboration, information sharing, and constantly monitoring the environment are fundamental tools in preventing catastrophes.

Whether the threat is natural, accidental, or intentional, identifying the threat, working to reduce vulnerabilities, and remaining prepared to recognize and act when the threat is in its earliest stages are all key to effective prevention. Implementation of this protocol is especially important in dealing with catastrophic threats.

Choosing where and when to intervene —and not intervene—are critical decisions. There are always too many threats to prevent every possibility. **Which potential catastrophes *must* we avoid?** Which threats are so horrible—and entirely possible—that an investment is required to prevent such outcomes?

Making these tough decisions, and the self-aware trade-offs that come with most tough decisions, is a big part of preventing catastrophe. Few right or wrong answers exist for this challenge. The decisions are mostly only better or worse. Constantly monitoring a range of threats and adjusting your decisions is necessary. The risk of catastrophe changes over time.

As with so much in fire service work, a persistent and disciplined approach to thinking and doing can achieve a great deal.

A Prevention Protocol

A protocol is a self-consciously disciplined approach to thinking and doing. It is a framework for working with a problem. A protocol does not provide an easy formula for making prevention decisions. It does offer a powerful way to consider problems using prevention principles.

Terrorists make strategic choices based on what they see as vulnerabilities. You can make choices that lessen vulnerabilities and identify the weaknesses of those attacking. Natural and accidental threats are broadly predictable. As such, you can identify vulnerabilities in advance and take action to reduce the level of vulnerability.

By applying a prevention protocol or framework to natural, accidental, and intentional threats, you are better able—especially when working with others—to identify those threats so potentially catastrophic that they require ongoing attention. In his classic manual for the London Fire Brigade, *A Complete Manual of the Organization, Machinery, Discipline, and General Working of the Fire Brigade of London* (1876), Sir Eyre Massey Shaw offered the following insight into the relationship between controlling a problem and developing new frameworks for thinking about the problem. "If you wish to control a problem, you must know more about the problem than anyone else and if you need to know more about the problem, you must

---

*A **protocol** is an organized and specifically structured way of behaving. It suggests a step-by-step process that is used again and again in a similar way. A protocol is often a set of rules to follow. Following the step-by-step process improves chances of achieving a desired outcome.*

What are some of the protocols most commonly used in the fire service?

Are there times when a protocol can complicate solving a problem? How do you decide when—or how—to apply a protocol?

_____
_____
_____
_____
_____
_____
_____
_____
_____
_____
_____
_____

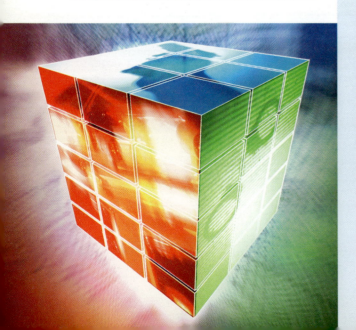

coin a terminology, a lexicon, that allows you to understand it." The prevention cube provides a terminology and unique conceptual framework for understanding the challenges faced in preparing for, and preventing, catastrophe.

The classic approach to Hazardous Materials planning includes identifying hazards, analyzing vulnerabilities, establishing priorities, assessing resources, and taking appropriate action (Plaugher). This is complementary to the five-step Prevention Protocol. The prevention protocol offered here visualizes the terms it uses as dimensions of a cube to facilitate thinking about the risks of catastrophe and preparing for it. The prevention cube provides a framework for fire service professionals to use in thinking about the problem of catastrophic risk, whether natural, accidental, or intentional. The prevention cube exemplifies relationships between factors in three ways.

The proactive and prevention-oriented principles of professional firefighters can support other public safety professions. For example, hazardous materials are "force multipliers" in natural, accidental, and intentional disasters. By tracking, understanding, sharing information, and managing the risk of hazardous materials, fire professionals move from first responders to first preventers.

Think of the relationships outlined by the prevention cube as rules of thumb for guiding prevention activities. They are arranged in a sequence. The **front face of the cube** shows five steps to enhance your ability to prevent a catastrophe.

- **Collaborate**
- **Share Information**
- **Recognize Threats**
- **Manage Risk**
- **Decide to Intervene**

This is the process for deciding where, when, and how to take action. Sometimes the process will happen in order—other times it might not.

Fire service personnel often rely on a combination of rule sets and professional intuition. Both of these come into play when people need to act quickly.

Professionals learn rule sets as a way to cultivate their intuition. Rule sets come from training and from understood roles and procedures. The life we lead when we are not in crisis influences our intuitions. We talk about intuition in terms of doing what we have to do, or doing the best we can. Intuition is part of being human. Intuition develops through experience and reflection.

The prevention cube is a way to combine the rules of prevention with your professional experience to face a variety of risks, and to distinguish between more ordinary risks and truly catastrophic risks.

THE PREVENTION CUBE:
Three Dimensions for Thinking and Acting

The **top** of the cube shows the three types of intervention:

- PROTECT – to physically or operationally "harden" a potential vulnerability
- DETER – to psychologically deter an intentional attack
- PREEMPT – to intervene sufficiently to interrupt an intentional attack or potential accident before it has had a full effect

The **front face** of the cube shows five steps to enhance your ability to prevent a catastrophe:

- COLLABORATE
- SHARE INFORMATION
- RECOGNIZE THREATS
- MANAGE RISK
- DECIDE TO INTERVENE

The **side** of the cube suggests that preventive action should be targeted for three distinct phases:

- PRIMARY – before a specific threat has emerged
- SECONDARY – when there are some early signals of a specific threat emerging
- TERTIARY – when a specific threat seems just about to occur

Social capital is the accumulation of good will, mutual trust, positive regard, and readiness to work together. In your fire service agency who has the most social capital with you? Why?

_____
_____
_____
_____
_____
_____
_____
_____
_____
_____
_____
_____

The Preparedness Professions

Responsibility for preventing catastrophe depends on law enforcement, the fire service, elected officials, emergency management, public health, public works, and many other public and private organizations.

Prevention methods are more effective if all preparedness professionals share them. Yet, each safety discipline has its own language, values and codes. "Stovepipes" divide prevention work according to job categories like police and fire, or state versus local authority. Preventing catastrophe depends on collaboration across stovepipes.

Saying that we want partnerships and trust building is one thing. Really doing it is another. The prevention cube is a shared framework that the several preparedness professions can use to talk together and put prevention into practice. Shared frameworks help everyone understand their roles, identify what they do best, decide where operational collaboration makes sense, and choose their priorities.

Collaborate

To collaborate is to plan, work, and exercise together to build trust and search for solutions to prevent catastrophes.

Collaboration goes beyond a single agency or department's point of view. Collaboration creates "social capital" and the awareness necessary to work the other steps in the prevention framework.

Collaboration is important early in the prevention process. By the time a crisis arrives, it is often too late to build relationships and trust. Building collaborative relationships leads to better information sharing, threat recognition, risk management and more opportunities for taking action. Collaboration increases intervention opportunities.

Share Information

To share information is to gather, store, analyze, distribute, and consume information and intelligence in order to prevent catastrophes.

Effective collaboration enables better information sharing. Preparedness professionals need to share information on threat identification, operations, and intelligence about potential threats and each profession's capabilities. They can also share information on vulnerabilities and on setting priorities. This kind of information sharing can help match a threat to a vulnerable target. Without information sharing and collaboration, each profession is more likely to be surprised and may not recognize an emerging threat until it is too late.

Recognize Threats

Recognizing specific natural, accidental, and intentional threats is a major goal for any collaborative process among _first preventers_.

A threat assessment identifies the potential of a threat given local historical patterns, recent trends beyond the locality, and the best information currently available.

Different disciplines tend to focus on different threats, though their concerns certainly go beyond any particular one.

- **Fire service professionals** focus largely on **ACCIDENTAL** and **INTENTIONAL THREATS**.
- **Police** tend to focus more on **INTENTIONAL THREATS**.
- **Emergency managers** and **public health officials** tend to focus on **NATURAL THREATS**.
- **Private sector** preparedness professionals traditionally are more concerned with **ACCIDENTAL THREATS**.

The prevention protocol offered here aims to enable *first preventers* to focus on the full spectrum of potential threats and vulnerabilities posing harm to their communities, thereby increasing the likelihood of recognizing the most dangerous threats and consequential vulnerabilities.

Manage Risks

To manage risk is to gauge the likelihood of specific threats and their potential impacts, including setting a minimum level of acceptable risk. Using risk management establishes a hierarchy of risk and balances threat, impact, and vulnerability, thereby minimizing the effects of an attack.

Vulnerability analysis identifies exploitable weaknesses. A vulnerability assessment can reveal flaws in security systems or water supplies, bridges, tunnels or other sensitive infrastructure. Risk analysis judges assets based on function. For example, power utilities, dams, and computer networks are different from sports stadiums and shopping malls.

While risk management benefits from several empirical tools, it remains an art and benefits from the considered judgment of various disciplines with varied experiences. Reasonable people will disagree. Especially when the goal is to prevent, or at least mitigate, a catastrophe, a collaborative process allows you to make the tough choices. Unless individuals and organizations perceive they have "ownership" of the risk management decision, they are unlikely to behave in accordance with the decision.

Decide to Intervene

Deciding to intervene involves a choice to use specific resources to protect, deter, or preempt. Intervention typically includes joint training, shared funding of activities, or sustained joint operations. It is impossible to intervene on every risk. Effective intervention to prevent a catastrophe is usually collaborative.

An effective decision is a precondition to an effective intervention. **A decision is a self-conscious choice to intervene in one way and not in another.** A decision involves communicating with others affected by the choices involved. A real decision ensures that resources and behavior align with the choices made. A decision requires monitoring the environment to assess the course of intervention and any unintended consequences.

In the case of intentional threats—and especially terrorism—your decision to intervene should recognize that once the decision is noted by those with an intention to harm, it will probably produce a change for which a new decision to intervene is needed.

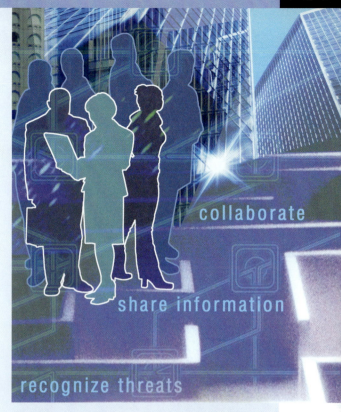

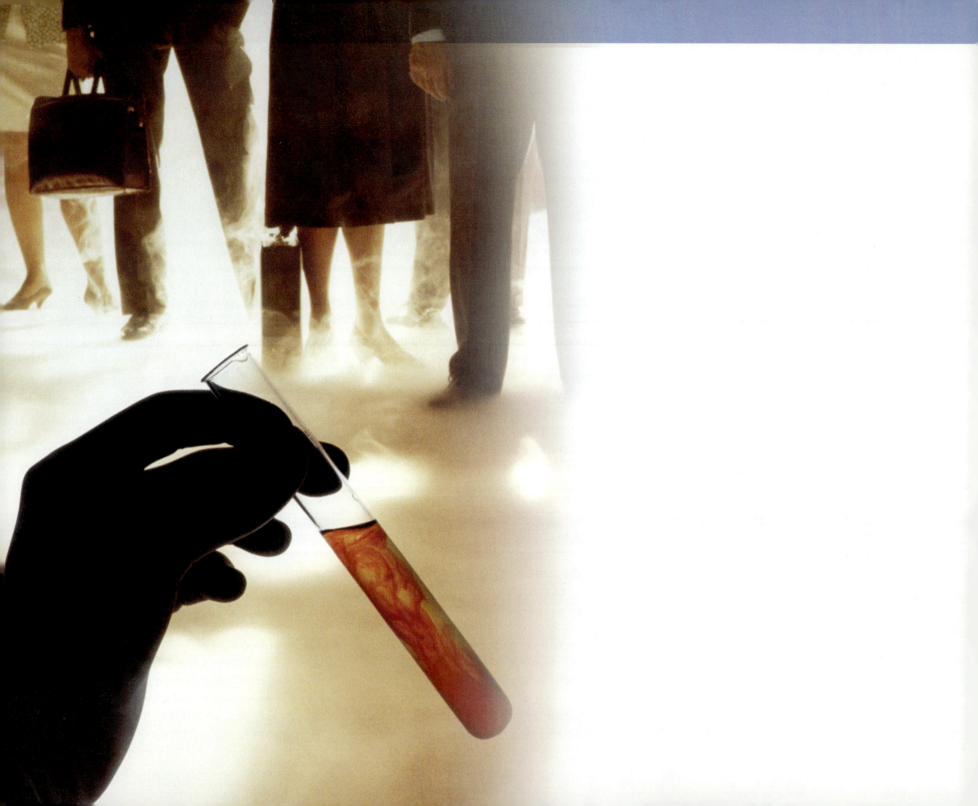

CHAPTER 1 — INTRODUCTION

INTENTIONAL THREATS: CHALLENGING OUR IMAGINATIONS

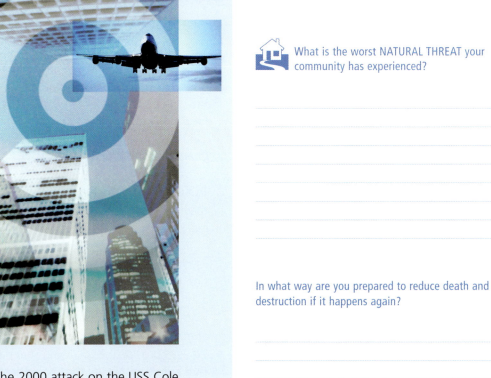

The *National Commission on Terrorist Attacks Upon the United States* found that our failure to prevent the September 11, 2001 attack was caused, in part, by **"a failure of imagination."**

The more time that passes without a subsequent serious attack, the more difficult it is to imagine the potential catastrophe of the next attack. The more time that passes, the easier it is to suppose that the attack will, at least, happen "somewhere else." The more time that passes, we are increasingly inclined to hope we have reduced the capacity of terrorists to launch serious—potentially catastrophic—attacks.

No one imagined the 1993 truck-bomb attack on the World Trade Center. No one imagined the 1995 bombing of the Murrah Federal Building in Oklahoma City. Why Oklahoma City? Did someone, other than the terrorists, imagine the sarin gas attack on the Tokyo subway? Did someone imagine a quiet city of 35,000 would be the target for a massacre of school children? Chechen terrorists probably chose Beslan as their target precisely because it seemed so unlikely. Who would have imagined an attack on two US embassies in East Africa on the same day in 1998? The 2000 attack on the USS Cole by what was nearly a rowboat is close to unimaginable—but it happened.

Terrorists depend on surprise. Terrorists want to keep our imaginations in low gear. The less we expect the attack, the more likely they are to succeed. The less we expect it, the more psychologically effective the result.

To prevent catastrophe, preparedness professionals need to consider natural, accidental, and intentional threats. Intentional threats, however, require some special attention because these threats complicate prevention through the terrorists' intention to mislead and surprise. As a result, much of the information and thinking offered herein, while

What is the worst NATURAL THREAT your community has experienced?

In what way are you prepared to reduce death and destruction if it happens again?

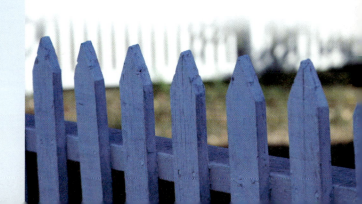

🏠 **What is the worst ACCIDENTAL THREAT your community has experienced?**

_____
_____
_____

Have you taken steps to reduce the chance it will happen again?

_____
_____
_____

Are there other likely sources of accidental disaster?

_____
_____
_____
_____
_____

What is the worst INTENTIONAL THREAT your community has experienced?

_____
_____
_____
_____
_____

What is the worst intentional threat for which your community is prepared?

_____
_____
_____
_____

sustaining a focus on all-hazards threat, aims to bolster your capability to imagine the conditions in your community that provide terrorists with opportunities to cause catastrophic harm.

Imagining the Worst

To prevent catastrophe you have to envision the catastrophic. You have to believe it is a real possibility. This is hard to do.

Psychologists have found that several decision-making habits discourage us from taking a long-term view, especially in regard to long-term threats. In their book *Predictable Surprises,* Max H. Bazerman and Michael D. Watkins provide the following summary of **five common biases that complicate our ability to prevent catastrophe:**

1. We tend to have **positive illusions** that lead us to conclude that a problem does not exist or is not severe enough to merit action.

2. We tend to **interpret events in an egocentric manner**. That is, when considering the fairness of proposed solutions to a looming crisis, we allocate credit and blame in ways that are self-serving.

3. We **overly discount the future**, reducing our courage to act now to prevent some disaster that we believe to be quite distant.

4. We tend to **maintain the status quo**, and refuse to accept any harm that would bring about a greater good. In other words we are reluctant to accept that some dramatic change will occur if we fail to address a mounting problem. Rather than confronting unpalatable choices, we avoid action altogether.

5. Most of us don't want to invest in **preventing a problem that we have not personally experienced or witnessed through vivid data**. Thus, far too often, we only fix problems after we ourselves experience significant harm or after we can clearly imagine ourselves, or those close to us, in peril.

The process built into the prevention cube helps overcome these built-in biases.

INTRODUCTION:
Chapter Review

Risk is the result of an interaction of **two factors**. What are those factors?

Risk = _____ x _____

This Workbook consistently references three **threat categories**. What are the three categories?

1 _____

2 _____

3 _____

How does a **catastrophe** differ from a crime, a disaster, or other such events?

_____
_____
_____
_____
_____
_____
_____
_____

Why is **prevention** especially important when dealing with the potential for a catastrophe?

_____
_____
_____
_____
_____
_____
_____
_____
_____
_____

Why are **intentional threats** especially difficult to predict (and therefore difficult to prevent)?

_____
_____
_____
_____
_____
_____

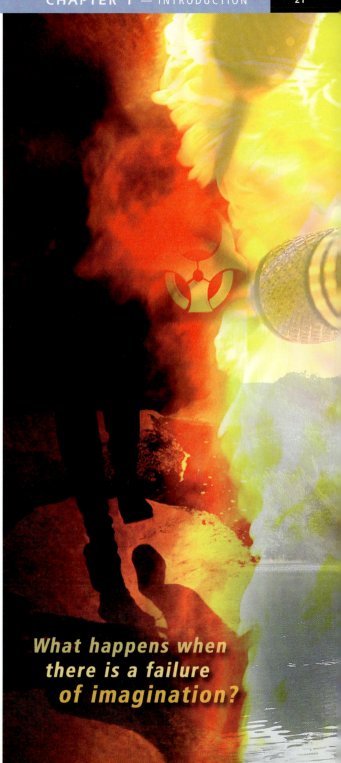

What happens when there is a failure of imagination?

APPLY WHAT YOU HAVE LEARNED

🔘 **Please use your CD to access the Terrorism Prevention Introductory Exercise.** Select the **Chapter 1** Certificate Course links located in the Online Exercises section of your CD.

In the exercise an attack on the fictional jurisdiction of San Luis Rey® may be imminent. **Can you apply a prevention protocol to this situation to successfully prevent an attack?**

To begin the exercise, you will select an avatar—in this case a Senior Captain in the San Luis Rey Fire Department. As you move through the prevention protocol steps, you will make choices, identify strategies, and work within the parameters of your selections and approaches. You have the opportunity to select collaborative partners and to determine an information-sharing approach to allow you access to certain pieces of information and deny you access to others. Based on your contacts and available information, you will try to identify emerging threats and manage the risks associated with individuals of concern and their capabilities.

Will you intervene? If so, how and with what level of aggression?

Fail and the consequences could be devastating.

Succeed and you are one step closer to understanding how to implement a prevention protocol in your own jurisdiction.

Note: If you have already enrolled in the Homeland Security Terrorism Prevention Certificate Course for Fire Service Professionals (©IPS) you can go directly to the exercise by typing this URL into your browser's address window:

www.preventivestrategies.net/game/mhfs-exercise

For first time access, use this initial URL:
www.preventivestrategies.net/go/mhfs-enroll

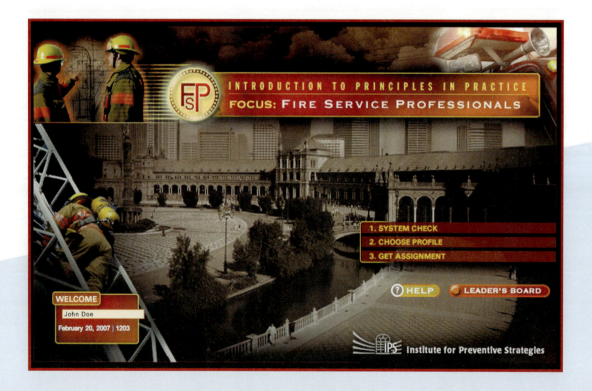

San Luis Rey® is a fictional jurisdiction designed by Teleologic Learning LLC.
All characters, locations, and events are fictitious and intended for instructional purposes only.

CHAPTER 1 — INTRODUCTION

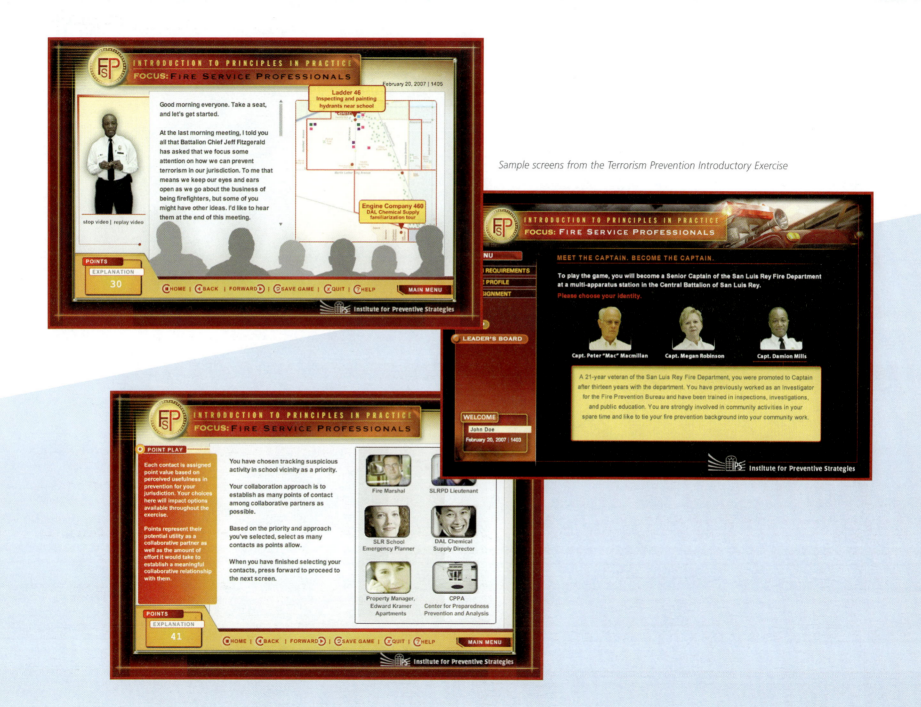

Sample screens from the Terrorism Prevention Introductory Exercise

How to Prevent Catastrophe

Recognize Threats
who and/or what? where are you most vulnerable?

Share Information
about who and what, and where you are most vulnerable

Collaborate
to share information, identify threats, share resources, plan, and train

Manage Risks
choose priorities and non-priorities

Decide to Intervene
communicate, coordinate, and follow-through

The first three steps of the prevention protocol can be swapped and switched. Where you begin depends on where you and others in *your* community are ready to begin. But whatever the first three steps, they lead to risk management and intervention decisions.

Recognize Threats

✓ *In this chapter you will learn:*

- **How to conduct a very basic threat assessment.**
- **How to distinguish between a catastrophic and a non-catastrophic threat.**
- **How vulnerability and threat relate to one another and influence both likelihood and consequences.**
- **How criticality is an important aspect of vulnerability and consequences.**
- **How psychological and social response to a disaster may be the crucial factor in determining whether or not it is a catastrophic event.**

The 9/11 Commission concluded that the events leading up to the terrorist attacks on September 11, 2001 resulted from a *lack of imagination* on the part of those whose mission is counterterrorism. Imagination is a crucial component in any strategy for recognizing catastrophic threat.

The Office of Domestic Preparedness, now referred to as the FEMA Training and Education Division (TED), in its 2003 *Guidelines for Homeland Security, Prevention and Deterrence* report proposed that all first responders need training to recognize "an inventory of behaviors and/or activities that constitute suspicious behavior likely to forewarn of a pending terrorism conspiracy or plot" (p. 20). We offer some useful lists of activities in Chapter 6 for members of the fire service to keep in mind when trying to recognize potential terrorist operations. As numerous fire service professionals note, the fire service needs an emphasis on training for preparedness and prevention of all threats (natural, accidental, and intentional) that equals the traditional emphasis on training for response and recovery.

A lack of imagination is not limited to catastrophes caused by intentional acts of terrorists. In considering threats, it is important to think in terms of **threat amplifiers**, regardless of the source of the threat, that triggers a harmful sequence of events, i.e. cascading failures. The challenges posed by terrorists aiming to do harm are especially difficult to anticipate due to their efforts to mislead about strategy, tactics, and targets. Nevertheless, an all-hazards strategy of prevention mitigates harmful consequences and produces greater resilience for communities even when terrorists succeed.

To help overcome an imagination-deficit, **try to think like a terrorist who is targeting your jurisdiction**.

What intentions would the terrorist bring to the task? What would the attack be meant to achieve? Who is the audience for the

Try to think like a terrorist who is targeting your jurisdiction. What intentions would the terrorist bring to the task?

What would the attack attempt to achieve?

Who is the audience for the attack?

What behavior is the attack meant to influence?

How would target selection be influenced by these intentions and purposes?

How would **local strengths and vulnerabilities** influence target selection? Can you develop a sympathetic imagination regarding terrorist motivations and goals?

Resilience is the ability to recover quickly.

CHAPTER 2 — RECOGNIZE THREATS

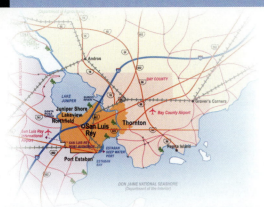

This workbook features examples and exercises from the fictional City of San Luis Rey. When you participate in the online exercises you become a member of the San Luis Rey Fire Department. **San Luis Rey is a fictional composite of many jurisdictions. Yet, each threat and vulnerability is based on a real-world situation somewhere in the United States.**

🔘 More information on San Luis Rey, including an introductory movie, is available on your CD.

San Luis Rey® is a registered service mark of Teleologic Learning LLC. **The "terrorist" portraits and descriptions at right are all fictional.**

IDEOLOGICAL TERRORISTS

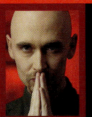

STEVE HACKETT

The American Christian Patriots Group in San Luis Rey gained momentum in the Spring of 2003 when Steve Hackett, a young charismatic deacon at the New Life Community Church and a vocal advocate for the right of self-segregation, assumed leadership of the local group. To fund activities in pursuit of a new order—one that ensures that the Jews and non-whites are not controlling their "earthbound and eternal destinies" and their ability to promote their children to their rightful places of leadership— Hackett joined other white supremacists across the state in political and fund-raising activities. These activities included protesting at abortion clinics across the state, allegedly participating in the planning of bank robberies, and attending state gun shows to accumulate the cache of weapons.

The core of the American Christian Patriots SLR group is 15 men in their early to mid-twenties. In May 2005, they launched a major recruiting effort in San Luis Rey, including the American Christian Patriots website and a newsletter (*ARISE*) which they distribute at places where groups of white young men gather.

RELIGIOUS TERRORISTS

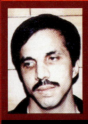

SAMI BASSEMI

Sami Bassemi, a Sunni Muslim, shares an apartment with three other men of Middle Eastern descent, Robert Farzid, 19, Abu Zarik, 22, and Mohammed Jidar, 24, in the Uptown District of San Luis Rey. They worship at Al Sabur Mosque. According to his visa, Sami is a student at San Luis Rey State University. University records show that he has not attended classes in over 18 months. Mr. Bassemi has organized a group of young men who congregate to study weaponry and tactics from US Army Manuals.

The group consists of men from varying backgrounds including second generation immigrants from several Islamic countries and American converts to Islam. The group meets at member's homes and at The Back Shed Gun Shop and Range with a virtual arsenal of weapons including rifles, shotguns, 9-mm and .357 caliber handguns, and AK-47 assault weapons. Many of the men have expressed sympathies with Islamic Fundamentalist jihadist causes, including those of Osama bin Laden.

TERRORIST CATEGORIES

attack? What behavior is the attack meant to influence?

How would target selection be influenced by these intentions and purposes? How would local strengths and vulnerabilities influence target selection? Can you develop a sympathetic imagination regarding terrorist motivations and goals?

🔘 To help imagine yourself as a terrorist, see *The Mind of a Terrorist* (Sauter and Carafano) on the CD provided with this workbook.

Depending on their motivations and objectives different terrorists will choose different targets and utilize different methods. **The more you understand the terrorist the more effectively you can prevent this intentional threat.**

🔘 Information on many terrorist organizations is available online. Use the reference library on the CD to access helpful websites.

Experts debate the readiness of terrorist organizations to conduct a catastrophic attack. Some argue that the most well organized terrorist organizations are especially sensitive to public opinion — meaning they would not risk a biological or radiological attack that their supporters might find offensive.

Others argue that, even if the moderating influence of public opinion on the most sophisticated terrorists is accepted, the proliferation of smaller, free-lance, and even more

CHAPTER 2 — RECOGNIZE THREATS

NATIONALIST TERRORISTS

RANDY McELROY

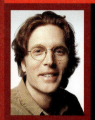

Randy McElroy is a founding member of The Serpent Dance Club. He is a research analyst at NGTT and lives in the Canal District. He has coordinated the group's travels to Northern Ireland and collected money for their charitable events.

The group was first formed during the World Cup soccer matches in 2002, when a contingent of young Irish fans gathered at The Serpent Dance Club to watch the Republic of Ireland matches. The participants are mostly male white-collar employees between twenty and thirty-five years of age. While the male members of the group are generally constant, attendance of the few female members is intermittent.

This group meets in small numbers on a regular basis. The Serpent Dance Club group has organized several charity events including a St. Patrick's Day 5-K, a small golf tournament, and a silent auction Christmas party at the club. The charity that was supported in each case was the Irish Republican Welfare Association (IRPWA). The U.S. Department of State identified the IRPWA as an alias for the Real Irish Republican Army (RIRA), a designated Foreign Terrorist Organization.

ISSUE ORIENTED TERRORISTS

LAUREN BOYD

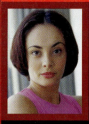

The Youth for Earth's Salvation (YES!) is a well-organized and well-publicized group founded by Lauren Boyd, a 2001 graduate from the San Luis Rey State University's (SLRSU) Master's Program in Political Science with a focus in communications (Radio/TV/Internet). Ms. Boyd founded the group in opposition to genetic research at the SLRSU's graduate agriculture program. Ms. Boyd now serves as the organization's Executive Director and sole employee. She has been arrested for trespassing at the Lake Juniper Water Authority Corporate Headquarters.

Due to Boyd's background, YES! is very media savvy and careful not to publicly call for violent activities to advance their political agenda. Their website, however, shows that YES! not only approves but is also supportive of such independent actions by its members. YES! is directly linked to People for the Ethical Treatment of Animals (PETA), an organization that has provided funding to the Earth Liberation Front (ELF), and indirectly linked to ELF itself.

TERRORIST CATEGORIES

Which of the terrorists shown at left is **most likely to threaten your community?**

_____
_____
_____
_____
_____
_____

radical groups increases the probability of terrorists seeking catastrophic results.

🌐 For more information on the possibility of a catastrophic attack on the United States please access the CD. A skeptical view of the threat is outlined by *Putting WMD Terrorism into Perspective* (Parachini). A more ominous analysis is offered in *All God's Poisons: Reevaluating the Threat of Religious Terrorism in regard to Non-Conventional Weapons* (Dolnik).

WHO AND/OR WHAT

Which of the terrorist types shown above and on the previous page is most likely to threaten your community?

There are several ways to categorize terrorists. This **four-part structure** is one of the most common:

- **IDEOLOGICAL TERRORISTS** are motivated to achieve a vision for their society reflected in a set of secular values and objectives that go beyond a single issue or identity group.

- **RELIGIOUS TERRORISTS** are also pursuing a vision for their society, but base that vision on a religious foundation.

- **NATIONALIST TERRORISTS** are generally fighting against what they perceive to be the oppression or marginalization of the ethnic, racial, or cultural group with which they identify. Nationalist terrorists may also claim ideological or religious motivation, but these values are used to support rather than motivate the terrorism.

- **ISSUE ORIENTED TERRORISTS** are focused on narrow special interests often involving a particular political policy. Once again religious or ideological values may be used to support the terrorism, but do not motivate it.

TERRORIST PROFILE

Select one terrorist organization that you consider a likely threat to your community.

💿 Utilize the web resources highlighted on the CD to research this type of terrorist. Based on what you discover, **develop a profile of the individual terrorist that you perceive as the most serious threat to your community.**

Answer the following as if you were that terrorist.

Your Age: _____

Your Level of Education: _____
_____

Your Special Skill: _____
_____

Your Personal Motivation (Why are you ready to cause harm to others?) _____
_____
_____

Your Organization's Motivation (Why does the organization perceive that causing harm to others is justified and/or effective?)
_____
_____
_____

Your Organization's Strategic Objective (What outcome is the organization attempting to achieve?)
_____
_____
_____

Does your organization seek to undertake a catastrophic attack? *(circle one)*

    Yes   No   Not sure

Does your organization have a **reasonable capacity** to undertake a catastrophic attack? *(circle one)*

    Yes   No   Not sure

Given the motivation, intention, and track record of your terrorist group, what do you consider the **most likely target in your community**? *(These categories are based on the Department of Homeland Security's Strategy and Assessment Tool-kit.)*

___ Real Estate Development
___ Agricultural Sector
___ Banking and Financial System
___ Civic and Social Institutions (including public symbols)
___ Commercial/Industrial Facilities
___ Electric Power System
___ Emergency Services
___ Government Services
___ Information/Communications (including telecommunications and computers)
___ Public Health
___ Recreational Facilities
___ Transportation Centers
___ Water Supply
___ Other, please specify: _____
_____

Is your above selection different if, instead of asking "most likely," you ask yourself **what target when successfully attacked results in the most *devastation*?**

_____

If a catastrophe is an event that "changes everything for always," would an effective attack on any particular target result in catastrophic damage?

_____

CHAPTER 2 — RECOGNIZE THREATS

Even if you consider such an attack unlikely, where would a successful attack produce the **broadest and longest-term impact**?

_____

Which **target**, if successfully attacked, would make **recovery** the most difficult?

_____

Given the motivation, intention, and track record of your terrorist group, what do you consider the *most likely* **method of attack in your community**? *(The following attack methods are based on several chapters in* Homeland Security, *by Sauter and Carafano.)*

___ Ambush
___ Assassination
___ Sabotage
___ Kidnapping
___ Hostage Taking
___ Antiaircraft Missiles
___ Hijackings
___ Bombings
___ Suicide Attacks
___ Hoax
___ Siege
___ Drive-by Shooting
___ High Yield Explosives (e.g. Murrah Federal Building and WTC 1993)
___ Chemical Weapons
___ Industrial Chemical Attack
___ Biological Attack on Food Supply
___ Biological Attack using Human Disease
___ Radiological Attack (Dirty Bomb)
___ Nuclear Attack (Stolen Weapon)
___ Attack on Nuclear Power Infrastructure
___ Cyber attack
___ Other, please specify: _____
_____

Is your selection different if, instead of asking "most likely," you ask yourself **what method of attack results in the most** *devastation*? Which of these methods strike you as **most catastrophic**?

_____
_____

Which **method**, if successfully utilized, makes **recovery** the most difficult?

_____
_____

By answering these Who and/or What questions you have conducted simple threat-based and capabilities-based threat assessments.

A threat-based approach focuses on a specific adversary. Knowing and monitoring a specific adversary is enormously helpful. However, in many cases the source of a potential intentional threat is unidentified. **As a result, it is often helpful to think in terms of attack capabilities rather than specific attackers.** Anticipating and reducing the likelihood of any specific capability is helpful regardless of who might attack. **Reducing vulnerability to intentional threats may also reduce vulnerability to natural and accidental threats.**

Consider the history of natural, accidental, and intentional threats in your community. Over the last twenty years which of these threats has caused the greatest difficulty?

_____
_____
_____
_____

Does your answer change if you look at the last century?

_____
_____
_____

Has your community experienced a catastrophic hurricane, flood, fire, or earthquake?

_____
_____
_____
_____

Has your community experienced a catastrophic accident—or an accident that was too close to catastrophe for comfort?

_____
_____
_____
_____

Can you find credible evidence of actual or planned intentional threats in your community?

_____
_____
_____
_____

YOUR LOCAL HISTORY

Now that you have imagined some possible intentional threats, consider the history of natural, accidental, and intentional threats in your community. Over the last twenty years which of these threats has caused the greatest difficulty? Does your answer change if you look at the last century?

Has your community experienced a catastrophic hurricane, flood, fire, or earthquake? Has your community experienced a catastrophic accident—or an accident that was too close to catastrophe for comfort? Can you find credible evidence of actual or planned intentional threats in your community?

Not every intentional threat is designed to incite terror, even under the current, fairly broad definition of terrorism. According to the *Uniting and Strengthening America by Providing Appropriate Tools Required to Intercept and Obstruct Terrorism* (USA PATRIOT) *Act* of 2001, and similar language used in other federal statutes, terrorist activities,

(A) involve acts dangerous to human life that are a violation of the criminal laws of the United States or of any State;
(B) appear to be intended—
   (i) to intimidate or coerce a civilian population;
   (ii) to influence the policy of a government by intimidation or coercion; or
   (iii) to affect the conduct of a government by mass destruction, assassination, or kidnapping…

If the intention behind criminal acts, planned or perpetrated, is aimed at political or social outcomes then a case can be made for terrorism under the US Code and several state statutes. For example, the assassination of doctors who perform abortions can be an illegal act designed to influence government policy. The kidnapping or murder of minority citizens has been used as a means of systematic coercion. Students planning to assault teachers and students have been charged with terrorism. The FBI tracks so-called eco-terrorists who use violence to protest or delay what they perceive as attacks on the environment.

You have already been introduced to a four-category framework for identifying terrorists: nationalist, religious, ideological, and special interests. The Southern Poverty Law Center's Intelligence Project uses a seven-category framework that focuses on prominent kinds of domestic terrorists:

- Black Separatist
- Ku Klux Klan
- Neo-Nazi
- Racist Skinhead
- Christian Identity
- Neo-Confederate
- Other (examples include the Jewish Defense League, Council of Conservative Citizens, and Women for Aryan Unity)

CHAPTER 2 — RECOGNIZE THREATS

Natural & Accidental Threats

Look again at the list of community assets below. Does your perception of vulnerability change depending on the kind of threat you anticipate?

_____
_____

Which of the following do you consider most vulnerable to a **NATURAL** threat?

___ Agricultural Sector
___ Banking and Financial System
___ Civic and Social Institutions (including public symbols)
___ Commercial/Industrial Facilities
___ Electric Power System
___ Emergency Services
___ Government Services
___ Information/Communications (including telecommunications and computers)
___ Public Health
___ Recreational Facilities
___ Transportation Centers
___ Water Supply
___ Lumber, Fishing, and Mining
___ Other, please specify: _____

Which are most vulnerable to an **ACCIDENTAL** threat?

___ Agricultural Sector
___ Banking and Financial System
___ Civic and Social Institutions (including public symbols)
___ Commercial/Industrial Facilities
___ Electric Power System
___ Emergency Services
___ Government Services
___ Information/Communications (including telecommunications and computers)
___ Public Health
___ Recreational Facilities
___ Transportation Centers
___ Water Supply
___ Lumber, Fishing, and Mining
___ Other, please specify: _____

How do these answers compare to the ranking you have already given for an intentional threat?

_____
_____

If you do not have sufficient information to make these judgments, how can you get good information?

_____
_____
_____

Patterns of Terrorist Behavior

Have you recently had or do you currently have evidence of planned violence that is consistent with patterns often characterized by terrorists?

_____
_____
_____
_____
_____
_____
_____
_____
_____
_____
_____
_____
_____
_____
_____
_____
_____
_____
_____

Carl Conetta, from the Project on Defense Alternatives, contends that terrorist groups generally engage in **three types of attacks:** instrumental, catalytic, and immanent.

An **Instrumental** strategy seeks an immediate gain or concession of some sort; or it seeks to deter some policy. A **Catalytic** strategy seeks to inspire a constituency or to provoke a broader confrontation. **Immanent** strategies are those in which terror and destruction seem to be ends in themselves—although the terrorist actor may see them as part of some greater plan.

Some argue that **immanent strategies include two important sub-categories**:

- **Apocalyptic terrorism:** a desperate act of defiance and protest; and
- **Expressive terrorism**: a blow against a social order that is regarded as corrupt beyond reform (sometimes also called **Nihilistic** terrorism).

While all of these threat patterns are worth serious attention, in considering catastrophic threat we should focus mostly on sources of catalytic and immanent, or grand, attacks. Al-Qaeda, for example, has encouraged its network and sympathizers to seek the "biggest bang for their buck" in planning the largest, most devastating attacks possible with the smallest possible investment of resources.

Many intentional threats are instrumental. These are certainly important issues of public safety. However, **to prevent and mitigate catastrophe, the most productive focus is on groups inclined toward catalytic and immanent strategies.**

WEAPONS OF CATASTROPHE

The legal definition of a Weapon of Mass Destruction encompasses something as small as a pipe bomb. In layman's terms—and in terms of preventing catastrophe—our WMD threats are more expansive. Some of the more dangerous are outlined below:

Toxin. Although a toxin is usually defined as a toxic substance produced by living organisms (e.g., animals, bacteria, fungi, plants), the U.S. is a signatory to both the Biological and Toxin Weapons Convention and the Chemical Weapons Convention. Under those treaties, toxins are defined as chemical or biological warfare agents regardless of whether the substances are natural or synthetic in origin.

Chemically-based WMDs utilize toxic agents, including sarin gas, nerve gas, mustard gas, ricin, and cyanide, that can kill or paralyze. Iraq used poison gas on civilian populations during the 1980s and 1990s. Chemical agents can damage the respiratory system, digestive system, eyes, brain, blood, skin, and other organs. Chemical agents could be used in large-scale warfare, but also could be released into the ventilation system of a large office building. The U.S. military field manual for treatment of chemical warfare casualties (Field Manual No. 8-285) defines a chemical agent as "a chemical substance which, because of its physiological, psychological, or pharmacological effects, is intended for use in military operations, to kill, seriously injure, or incapacitate humans (or animals) through its toxicological effects. Excluded are riot control agents, chemical herbicides, and smoke and flame materials. Chemical agents are nerve agents, incapacitating agents, blister agents (vesicants), lung-damaging agents, blood agents and vomiting agents."

Biologically-based WMDs utilize bacterial or viral organisms—such as anthrax or smallpox—to infect populations (or the food chain) with diseases. According to the Center for Strategic and International Studies, "pounds or possibly ounces of a biological agent can do a job that would require tons of a chemical agent." These agents can be released into the air, water, or food supply. The U.S. Army defines biological agents as "living organisms, or the materials derived from them, that cause disease in, or harm, humans, animals, or plants, or cause deterioration of material. Biological agents may be found as liquid droplets, aerosols, or dry powders. A biological agent can be adapted and used as a terrorist weapon, such as anthrax, tularemia, cholera, encephalitis, plague, and botulism. There are three different types of biological agents: bacteria, viruses, and toxins." Similarly, so-called Category A weapons (the most dangerous or likely to be used by terrorists according to the Centers for Disease Control and Prevention) are anthrax, botulinum toxin, plague, ricin, smallpox, tularemia, and viral hemorrhagic fevers.

Radiological WMDs, radiological dispersal devices, radiological dispersal weapons, otherwise known as "dirty bombs," are explosive devices, including bombs or artillery shells, that spread radioactive materials generally in areas of high population density. For example, 3.5 ounces of plutonium could prove lethal to those in a large office building or factory. An attack with a dirty bomb could result in the contamination of persons, livestock, and food and water. Covert attacks could result in gradual radiation poisoning.

Nuclear WMDs including atom bombs, hydrogen bombs, and even small nuclear weapons (such as suitcase bombs) pose a grave threat both from the initial blast and the subsequent fallout. Delivery systems are usually ballistic missiles or bombs dropped by planes but a nuclear warhead could actually fit into a car or truck. On the other hand, access to essential elements such as plutonium and highly enriched uranium is difficult and expensive. Traditional nuclear weapons aren't the only threat; nuclear reactor sabotage or a reactor-core meltdown could release large amounts of radioactivity into the environment.

Historically, terrorists have operated with a conventional tactical inventory, using guns, knives, and bombs. Most terrorist incidents have involved bombings, assassinations, kidnappings, armed assaults, hostage situations, and hijacking. The 9/11 hijackers used boxcutters to take over the planes that struck the WTC and Pentagon. Subsequently, a terrorist tried to use a primitive shoe bomb on an American Airlines flight from Paris. Some argue that terrorists will most likely continue using conventional weapons.

Most predict that it is only a question of time before terror groups launch an attack within our borders using chemical, biological, radiological, or nuclear (i.e., CBRN), or high-yield explosive weapons. Former President Clinton has said **there is a 100 percent chance of a chemical or biological attack on U.S. soil within the next ten years.**

The *National Strategy for Combating Terrorism* defines the terrorist acquisition and use of WMDs as a "clear and present danger," and that "a central goal [of the strategy] must be to prevent terrorists from acquiring or manufacturing the WMD that would enable them to act on their worst ambitions."

This threat is underscored by the Health Physics Society, a nonprofit scientific professional organization that promotes radiation safety. **A WMD "can be anything from a simple child's balloon filled with a deadly toxin** or disease organism which can be burst over a crowd, to a 55-gallon drum filled with high explosives wrapped with radioactive material, a fully functional nuclear weapon, or anything in between. In short, it is impossible to detect a WMD device unless a responder has proper training, proper equipment, and some forewarning."

The U.S. Defense Department defines a WMD as any weapon or device intended, or having the capability of, causing death or serious bodily injury to a significant number of people through the release of toxic or poisonous chemicals or their precursors, a disease organism, or radiation or radioactivity. This includes detonating a nuclear weapon, or dispersing radioactivity, or chemical or biological agents via explosion, spraying, water supply contamination, or other "vectors."

 Further information is available on the CD in the reading: *Weapons of Mass Destruction: Understanding the Great Terrorist Threats and Getting Beyond the Hype* (Sauter and Carafano).

CHAPTER 2 — RECOGNIZE THREATS

Does your community provide access to any of the ingredients for the weapons of catastrophe listed on the previous pages? (circle one)

yes   no   I don't know

If YES, which ones?

_____
_____
_____
_____
_____

How **secure** are these local sources?

very secure   secure   not secure   I don't know

(Many of the sources are in the private sector. As a result fire service professionals in most jurisdictions are likely to answer, "I don't know." If you can answer confidently you are already well above the curve.)

Is there currently a method for **tracking any significant changes** in public access or utilization of the weapon sources outlined?

yes   no   I don't know

Are you familiar with signs and signals that the sources outlined above might be present in an unusual or suspicious setting?

yes   no

Do you know where to find out more about signs and signals of these sources?

yes   no

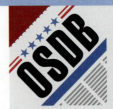

Open Source Daily Brief
BRIEF OF THE DAY (2006-09-29):
DHS Receives Authorization to Regulate High-Risk Chemical Facilities

The critical infrastructure of most countries, especially the United States, is the key to the functioning of basic economic, social, and political institutions. Homeland Security Presidential Directive 7 (HSPD-7), "Critical Infrastructure Identification, Prioritization, and Protection," released on December 17, 2003, outlined protection needs for the Nation's critical infrastructure. Companies in the private sector own most of the critical infrastructure in the United States. A key question facing proponents of securing critical infrastructure is whether the United States needs additional government regulations to ensure adequate safeguards against terrorist attack.

In the absence of federal regulations relating to threats against specific sectors of critical infrastructure, some states passed their own security regulations. Illinois, for example, stipulated security standards for its public utilities to follow last year. New Jersey took steps late last year to mandate security requirements for the chemical industry. Additionally, the Director of Homeland Security for New Jersey, Richard Canas, recently announced the state is considering using teams of undercover agents, or outside contractors, as "red teams" to test the security at New Jersey hospitals and chemical plants.

Earlier this year, the General Accountability Office (GAO) released a report that assessed the lead role taken by the Department of Homeland Security (DHS) in developing a Chemical Sector-Specific Plan intended to protect the chemical industry. The GAO study recommended that Congress give DHS the authority to address plant security in the chemical industry, among other recommendations. Until recently, the chemical industry generally opposed federal regulations regarding protection of its facilities.

Earlier this week the Senate and House agreed to provide DHS with oversight authority for high-risk chemical facilities. The National Petrochemical & Refiners Association responded to the new authority provided DHS by Congress as follows: "NPRA is pleased that the legislation recognizes the importance of protecting vulnerability assessments and specific site security plans from unwarranted and problematic public disclosure, as does the MTSA [Maritime Transportation Security Act]. The measure does provide for the appropriate sharing of information with state and local law enforcement officials, along with first responders, whose vital duties may require in-depth knowledge of security-related information."

PREVENTION RELEVANCE: A terrorist attack at chemical storage facilities could release a toxic cloud endangering surrounding communities for miles.

PREVENTION TECHNIQUES: Authorize the Secretary of Homeland Security to regulate high-risk chemical facilities.

PREVENTION THOUGHT: Risk Management
Do you support providing DHS with the authority to regulate the security of high-risk chemical facilities in the private sector?

The Open Source Daily Brief is a service of the Institute for Preventive Strategies (©IPS). You can register to receive the OSDBs at www.preventivestrategies.net.

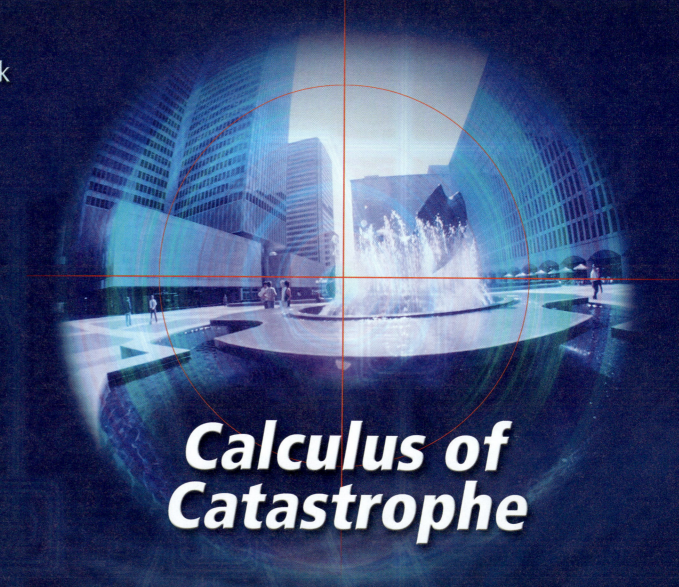

Terrorists seek to **multiply** their threat by exploiting your vulnerabilty.

You want to **divide** their threat by reducing your vulnerability.

Calculus of Catastrophe

Likelihood x Consequences = Risk

Likelihood = Threat { x **Vulnerability** if *(state conditions)*
/ **Vulnerability** if *(state conditions)*

CHAPTER 2 — RECOGNIZE THREATS

Risk = Likelihood x Consequences

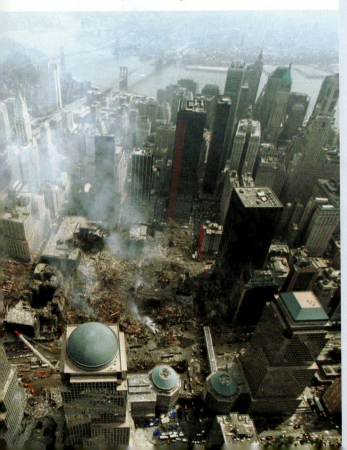

The smoldering site of the World Trade Center towers after 9/11, New York City, 2001. Source: U.S. Customs

VULNERABILITY

In the simple definition of risk previously provided, **Risk = Likelihood x Consequences**, **Likelihood** is determined by:

- **The presence of a threat**
- **The capabilities of a threat**
- **Visibility of targets**
- **Accessibility of targets**
- **Criticality of targets**

Visibility, accessibility and criticality are all key aspects of vulnerability.

When dealing with intentional threats, vulnerability can be something that is attractive to attack. A **target's attractiveness** depends on the intention of those attacking as well as the inherent strength or weakness of the target.

Anti-abortion terrorists tend to focus on abortion providers. Eco-terrorists focus on the logging and construction industries. Animal rights terrorists concentrate on the use of animals in pharmaceutical research and by the fashion industry. Al-Qaeda and its sympathizers attack military, political, and economic targets. Al-Qaeda has articulated a strategy to undermine the economic advantages of the United States and the West.

The World Trade Center towers were highly visible, reasonably accessible, and perceived to play a critical role in the US and international economies. The terrorists may have, in fact, over-estimated the practical criticality of the target. It is also possible that the WTC towers, Pentagon, and Capitol Building (probable target of the plane downed in Pennsylvania) were selected for symbolic purposes.

Many scholars of terrorism consider an intentional catastrophic attack unlikely. They argue using a weapon of catastrophe is not in the self-interest of the most capable terrorist organizations. Those organizations that might be most motivated to such an attack, they suggest, are unlikely to have sufficient sophistication and resources to carry out such an attack.

Jonathan B. Tucker of the Center for Nonproliferation Studies has found, "Motivations for the terrorist use of chemical, biological, radiologic, or nuclear materials appear to encompass a wide range of objectives…
1) to promote nationalist or separatist objectives;
2) to retaliate or take revenge for a real or perceived injury;
3) to protest government policies; and
4) to defend animal rights."

Yet, in the cases documented by Tucker, the terrorists' use of weapons of catastrophe remained limited, and did not produce catastrophic results.

Tucker and others note that **terrorist groups with a religiously based apocalyptic**

worldview may be the most likely to seek a catastrophe. There is also concern that an intended limited attack using a weapon of catastrophe could accidentally produce a much greater impact. A biological attack spreading more quickly and widely than anticipated is an example.

Vulnerability to Natural and Accidental Threats

In April 1906 San Francisco survived the big earthquake reasonably well. But the fire caused by the earthquake destroyed much of the city and made recovery much more difficult.

In August 2003 a series of natural and accidental threats interacted to black out electricity across much of the Midwest, Northeast, and Southern Canada. The electrical grid essentially collapsed. Over 50 million people were without power, some for nearly three days.

In September 2005 it initially seemed that New Orleans had avoided the worst, but the after-effects of the storm on the levees produced a true catastrophe.

What often transforms a disaster into a catastrophe is when a natural event encounters human failure. The interaction amplifies the original threat and associated cascading failures result in large-scale harm.

Many of these interactions can be imagined, but they are very difficult to precisely predict. Which combination of natural and accidental threats poses the biggest threat? Which combination is most likely?

Reduce Vulnerability

Most natural threats are not preventable, but vulnerability to the natural threats is reducible, and the outcomes mitigated by conscious choices taken in advance. Not all accidental threats are preventable, but decisions can reduce vulnerability to catastrophic consequences. Even if most intentional threats are preventable, just one successful attack using a weapon of catastrophe can produce profound harm.

Ignoring vulnerabilities multiplies the power of the threat. Dealing with vulnerabilities creatively and proactively can divide the power of the threat.

Likelihood x **Consequences** = **Risk**

Likelihood = **Threat** { x *Vulnerability if* (state conditions)
 / *Vulnerability if* (state conditions)

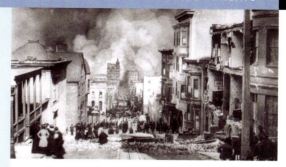

Devastating fires in San Francisco following the earthquake of 1906 (from the Steinbrugge Collection of the UC Berkeley Earthquake Engineering Research Center).

Which combination of natural and accidental threats poses the **biggest threat**?

Which combination is **most likely**?

Which combination of threats is most likely in your community?

How are the **ASSET-based and GEOGRAPHIC-based risk analysis models** the same as the simple methods already outlined? How do these models differ?

_____
_____
_____
_____
_____
_____
_____
_____
_____
_____
_____
_____

Which risk analysis model do you perceive is best suited for your community?

_____
_____
_____
_____
_____
_____
_____

A DHS Approach

The Department of Homeland Security's Urban Area Security Initiative (UASI) program utilizes two risk analysis models: **Asset-based** and **Geographic-based**.

The inputs used by the Asset-Based model will be similar for most communities. Each community will have very different outputs, but the data sources are relevant to most places. Look carefully at the inputs used to determine the Threat level in the Geographic model. What inputs would be better to use for your community?

A complete description of these methods is available on the CD. Following are visual representations of the two methods.

How are these models the same as the simple methods already outlined? How do these models differ? Which model do you perceive is best suited for your community?

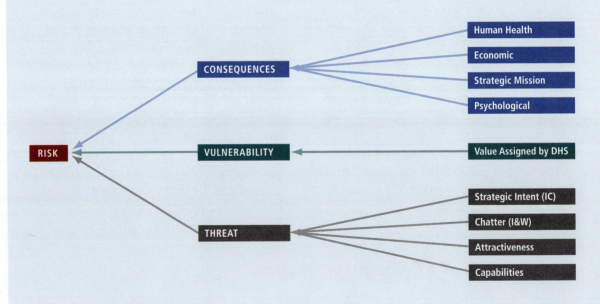

UASI Asset-Based Risk Analysis

CHAPTER 2 — RECOGNIZE THREATS

UASI Geographic Risk Analysis

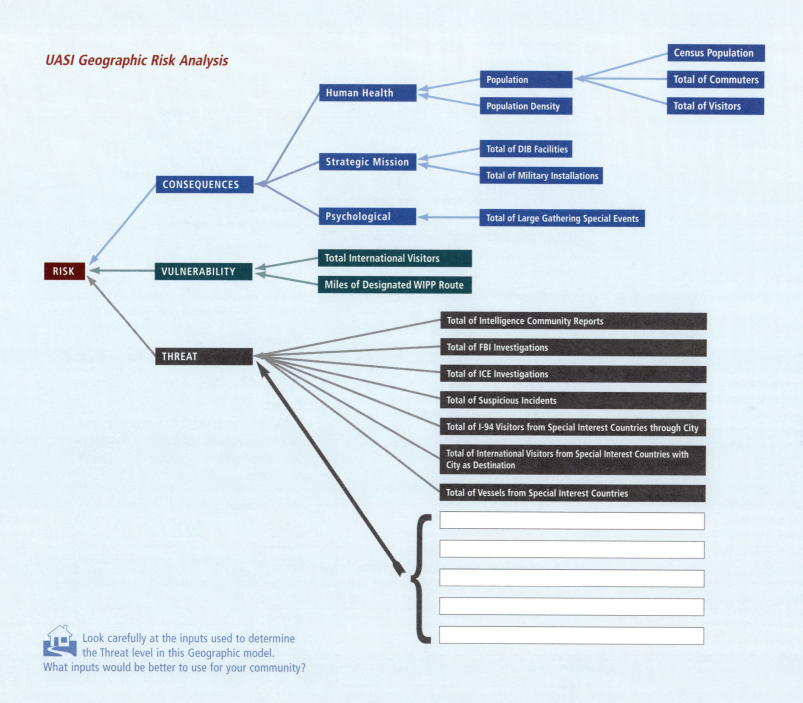

Look carefully at the inputs used to determine the Threat level in this Geographic model. What inputs would be better to use for your community?

CHAPTER 2 — RECOGNIZE THREATS

🏠 Which of the following **CRITICAL ASSETS** do you consider **most critical to the survival of your jurisdiction?** Rank order the five most important.

___ water supply
___ food supply
___ waste and sanitation services
___ sewage treatment
___ public health
___ primary health care
___ emergency health care
___ long-term and geriatric health care
___ housing supply
___ electricity supply
___ natural gas supply
___ gasoline supply
___ continuity of government
___ police services
___ public works services
___ fire services
___ judicial services
___ taxation and public revenue
___ rail transportation system
___ road transportation system
___ air transportation system
___ water transportation system
___ telephone communications
___ radio broadcasting
___ television broadcasting
___ Internet
___ commercial (wholesale and retail) sector
___ manufacturing sector
___ financial services sector
___ professional services sector
___ distribution sector
___ hospitality sector
___ public schools
___ colleges and universities
___ sports events
___ religious events
___ cultural events
___ political events
___ other: _____

Criticality as a Key Criterion of Vulnerability

Given the varied terrorist capabilities and the unpredictable interplay of natural and accidental threats, it is usually **more helpful to focus on criticality** rather than visibility or accessibility as the key aspect of vulnerability.

John Moteff of the Congressional Research Service has written, "Criticality is typically defined as a measure of the consequences associated with the loss or degradation of a particular asset. The more the loss of an asset threatens the survival or viability of its owners, of those located nearby, or of others who depend on it (including the nation as a whole), the more critical it becomes."

🏠 How many of the critical assets listed at left are actually located within your community? How can you reduce your community's vulnerability if the asset is outside your community?

_____
_____
_____

How many of these critical assets are privately owned? How can you reduce your community's vulnerability if the asset is privately owned?

_____
_____
_____

One common approach to vulnerability analysis is the **CARVER method**:

Criticality
What are your key nodes, choke points, and potential causes of cascading failure?

Accessibility
How easy is it for a threat to access or impact a critical asset?

Recoverability
How much time and money would be required to replace or restore a critical asset?

Vulnerability
Are there effective methods for securing the critical asset?

Effect
What are the adverse consequences that would result from a successful natural or accidental or intentional threat aimed at the critical asset?

Recognizability
What is the likelihood that an adversary will recognize the critical nature of the asset? Natural and accidental threats are more random, but terrorists recognize and consciously choose.

Each factor in CARVER is evaluated on a ten-point scale. The **CARVER + Shock** method is a variation on CARVER. It adds a seventh factor, **Shock**, that evaluates the combined health, economic, and psychological impacts of an attack, or the shock attributes of a target. (*CARVER Plus Shock Method…*)

Does your rank order of critical assets change if, instead of survivability, you are asked to identify those of most importance to **short-term recovery** (the first three weeks after a natural, accidental, or intentional catastrophe)?

Does your rank order change if you are asked to identify those of most importance to **long-term recovery** (one to three years after a natural, accidental, or intentional catastrophe)?

Are there **critical interdependencies** between these various elements? (For example food supply is probably dependent on some elements of the transportation system.) If so, how does this impact your rank ordering? In the case of your jurisdiction is the food supply best ensured by, for example, stockpiling or keeping open transportation links?

There are tools, protocols, and methods that can be used to organize effective vulnerability assessments. On the following page is a *Basic Vulnerability Assessment Worksheet* developed by the Department of Homeland Security. Such disciplined processes can contribute a great deal to thinking about and reaching well-informed decisions.

However, vulnerability assessment, criticality assessment, and other elements of risk analysis involve human judgments that are seldom reducible to an "expert system" or automated decision-making tool. Local conditions are too varied. The judgments involved are usually not black and white. Tough choices are required.

Outsourcing the tough choices to consultants is not a viable option in most circumstances. Involvement by those who have to live with the results is not optional. Those expected to implement the decisions must demand involvement in the decision-making. Outside consultants may play an important role in forcing insiders to examine uncomfortable facts. A small team may need to develop options for a larger group to examine. Yet, in preparing for catastrophe, a broad-based process of threat identification is the only process likely to produce actionable results.

It is difficult to imagine any sizable community without all of the sectors and services suggested by the list on the previous page. **But if everything is critical, nothing is critical.** To prepare for catastrophe it is necessary to choose what must be protected or quickly recoverable even if everything else is lost.

Review your list on the previous page. Does your rank order change if, instead of survivability, you are asked to identify those of most importance to **short-term recovery** (the first three weeks after a natural, accidental, or intentional catastrophe)?

_____
_____
_____

Does your rank order change if you are asked to identify those of most importance to **long-term recovery** (one to three years after a natural, accidental, or intentional catastrophe)?

_____
_____
_____

Are there **critical interdependencies** between these various elements? If so, how does this impact your rank ordering?

_____
_____
_____

In the case of your jurisdiction is the food supply best ensured by, for example, stockpiling or keeping open transportation links?

_____
_____
_____

CHAPTER 2 — RECOGNIZE THREATS

BASIC VULNERABILITY ASSESSMENT WORKSHEET

Complete the form for each of the five community elements that you identified as being most important to the survival of your community.

(Duplicate the form for each potential target.)

Target Name or Number:	Total Score Rating:	
Duplicate this form and use one for each potential target.		Value
1. Level of Visibility: Assess the awareness of the existence and visibility of the target to the general public. **0=Invisible:** Existence secret/Classified location **3=Medium Visibility:** Existence known locally **1=Very Low Visibility:** Existence not publicized **4=High Visibility:** Existence known regionally **2=Low Visibility:** Existence public but not well known **5=Very High Visibility:** Existence known nationally		
2. Criticality of Target Site to Jurisdiction: Assess usefulness of assets to local population, economy, government, etc. Potential targets deemed essential to the continuity of the jurisdiction. **0** = No usefulness **2** = Moderate usefulness **4** = Highly useful **1** = Minor usefulness **3** = Significant usefulness **5** = Critical		
3. Impact Outside the Jurisdiction: Assess the effect loss will have outside of the jurisdiction. **0** = None **2** = Low **4** = High **1** = Very Low **3** = Medium **5** = Very High		
4. PTE Access to Target: Assess the availability of the target for ingress and egress by a PTE (Potential Threat Element). **0 = Restricted:** Security patrol 24/7, fenced, alarmed, CCTV, controlled access requiring prior clearance, designated parking, no unauthorized vehicle parking within 300 feet of facility, protected air/consumable entry. **1 = Controlled:** Security patrol 24/7, fenced, alarmed, controlled access of vehicles and personnel, designated parking, no unauthorized vehicle parking within 300 feet of facility, protected air/consumable entry. **2 = Limited:** Security guard at main entrance during business hours, fenced, alarmed, controlled access of visitors, designated parking, no unauthorized vehicles parking within 300 feet of facility, protected air/consumable entry. **3 = Moderate:** Controlled access of visitors, alarmed after business hours, protected air/consumable entry, designated parking, no unauthorized vehicle parking within 50 feet. **4 = Open:** Open access during business hours, locked during non-business hours, unprotected air/consumable entry. **5 = Unlimited:** Open access, unprotected air/consumable entry		
5. Potential Target Threat of Hazard: Assess the presence of legal WMD material (CBRNE) in quantities that could be the target of a terrorist attack or would complicate the response to an incident at that facility. **0 = None:** No WMD materials present **1 = Minimal:** WMD materials present in moderate quantities, under positive control, and in secured locations. **2 = Low:** WMD materials present in moderate quantities and controlled. **3 = Moderate:** Major concentrations of WMD materials that have established control features and are secured in the site. **4 = High:** Major concentrations of WMD materials that have moderate control features. **5 = Very High:** Major concentrations of WMD materials that are accessible to non-staff personnel.		
6. Potential Target Site Population Capacity: Assess the maximum number of individuals at a site at any given time. **0** = 0 **2** = 251-5000 **4** = 15,001-50,000 **1** = 1-250 **3** = 5,001-15,000 **5** = >50,001		
7. Potential for Collateral Mass Casualties: Assess potential collateral mass casualties within a one-mile radius of the target site. **0** = 0-100 **2** = 251-5000 **4** = 15,001-50,000 **1** = 101-250 **3** = 5,001-15,000 **5** = >50,001		
TOTAL		
Basic Target Vulnerability Assessment Rating: Convert total score to a rating number from 1-12 using the following key. Transfer final rating to top right hand box in this form. 0 - 2 pts. = 1 9-11 pts. = 4 18-20 pts. = 7 27-29 pts. = 10 3 - 5 pts. = 2 12-14 pts. = 5 21-23 pts. = 8 30-32 pts. = 11 6 - 8 pts. = 3 15-17 pts. = 6 24-26 pts. = 9 33-35 pts. = 12		

SOURCE: *Reference Handbook*, U.S. Department of Homeland Security (DHS), Office for Domestic Preparedness (ODP)

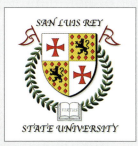

EXECUTIVE SUMMARY
OF THE SAN LUIS REY VULNERABILITY ANALYSIS

GRADUATE SCHOOL OF BUSINESS, SAN LUIS REY STATE

San Luis Rey® is a fictional jurisdiction designed by Teleologic Learning LLC. All characters, locations, and events are fictitious and intended for instructional purposes only.

This analysis seeks to identify critical areas of our city that possess attributes to make them both attractive to terrorist activity and vulnerable to terrorist attack. The analysis is organized around the three strategic objectives of the National Strategy for Homeland Security (July 2002).

STRATEGIC OBJECTIVE I: PREVENT TERRORIST ATTACK

The role of preventing terrorism falls largely on law enforcement and companies assigned to provide security to key assets. The current level of cooperation between local law enforcement agencies and federal law enforcement is poor. The dissemination of information regarding potential terrorist threats to the front line officers is also lacking. No formal relationship between the law enforcement community and private security teams charged with protecting private sector assets exists.

The prevention of bio-chemical attack focuses on the prevention of the introduction of, or the creation of, the means for such an attack. Related vulnerabilities that require a full security review include: the water purification and pumping stations, food processing centers, mail and parcel handling centers (outside the United States Postal Service).

STRATEGIC OBJECTIVE II: REDUCE OUR VULNERABILITY TO TERRORISM

San Luis Rey's critical infrastructure contains many segmented, independent, interrelated, public and private critical asset holders. Each piece of the critical infrastructure has its own independent security issues that must be addressed. In addition, the network itself also has specific security needs. To date, there has not been a full accounting of all elements of the critical infrastructure nor a written understanding of the interdependencies between these critical asset holders. Without both a clear roster of critical assets as well as a full understanding of their interdependent relationships, the assessment of vulnerability is incomplete.

STRATEGIC OBJECTIVE III: MINIMIZE THE DAMAGE AND RECOVER FROM TERRORIST ATTACKS

The current emergency management plan of San Luis Rey does not contemplate the loss of the entire municipal government complex as well as the loss of significant municipal employees and public office holders. The plan is also missing significant coordination and communication between emergency medical and mortuary facilities. In addition, the plan lacks a regional orientation in dealing with command and control, communications, emergency preparedness, training and exercising.

CONCLUSION:

The majority of the vulnerabilities exposed by this analysis are the result of advancing technologies, evolving threats and the regional impact of terrorist attacks. Any solutions designed to address these vulnerabilities should consider regional cooperation on all levels of government to be a top priority. Finally, vulnerability analysis is a dynamic process and should be regularly engaged to ensure that resources are being properly allocated to prevent attacks, reduce vulnerabilities, and minimize damage for a swifter recovery.

The full San Luis Rey Vulnerability report, available on the CD, more fully discusses vulnerabilities in four operational domains—Kinesthetic, Bio-Chemical, Cyber, and Public Confidence.

CHAPTER 2 — RECOGNIZE THREATS

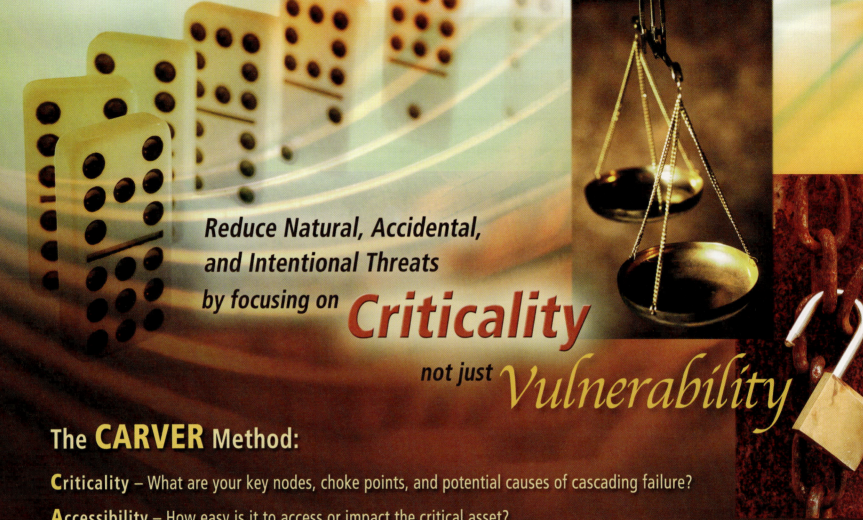

Reduce Natural, Accidental, and Intentional Threats by focusing on **Criticality** *not just* **Vulnerability**

The CARVER Method:

Criticality – What are your key nodes, choke points, and potential causes of cascading failure?

Accessibility – How easy is it to access or impact the critical asset?

Recoverability – How much time and money would be required to replace or restore a critical asset?

Vulnerability – Are there effective methods for securing the critical asset?

Effect – What are the adverse consequences that would result from a successful natural or accidental or intentional threat aimed at the critical asset?

Recognizability – What is the likelihood that terrorists will recognize the critical nature of the asset?

CONSEQUENCES

Likelihood, threat capabilities, vulnerability, and criticality are important factors in seeking to prevent or mitigate any threat. Yet, what most often distinguishes a catastrophic threat from other threats is in the **nature of the consequences.**

Several societies have survived—and even thrived—while dealing with an active intentional threat. Spain has made progress economically and politically despite Basque nationalist terrorism. Israel suffers sustained intentional threats but, so far, the consequences are such that something close to "normal" political, economic, and social life continues.

The March 11, 2004 terrorist bombing of Madrid commuter trains killed 191 and wounded over 1800. Many believe this attack also resulted in the Spanish ruling party losing a national election. The results of the attack were calamitous for the families affected. The political results were potentially very troublesome. Nevertheless, by most measures the consequences were less than catastrophic.

The DHS Vulnerability Assessment Worksheet shown on page 42 is biased toward "kinetic" attacks (usually bombs) on structures or events in a densely populated area. Given the prior pattern of terrorist attacks this is a reasonable bias. The 9/11 attacks, Madrid train bombing, and London commuter attacks, for example, were all kinetic. Was each event a catastrophe? If so, in what way and for whom? If not, why not?

Was the 1906 San Francisco earthquake a catastrophe? Was the 1997 Red River Flood and Grand Forks Fire a catastrophe? Was the 1991 Oakland Hills Fire a catastrophe? If so, in what way and for whom? If not, why not?

If a catastrophe is something from which recovery is nearly impossible, then the direct effects must be very broad and deep. The successful use of a dirty bomb in a major urban area would be a local catastrophe, potentially producing a dead zone unusable for more than a generation. But the direct impact on the nation could be less than catastrophic.

Would the simultaneous use of a dirty bomb in three urban centers be a national catastrophe or three local catastrophes? A significant radiological event in Washington D.C. could have a catastrophic impact far beyond the physical area directly affected.

Whether an event is catastrophic or not depends, in part, on **how society responds** to the event. We now know that the response to the 9/11 attacks—fear of flying, for example—produced an indirect economic impact that was much worse than the damage done by the attack itself. For the air passenger industry 9/11 changed everything. We are reminded of the changes each time we go through security to catch a flight.

Consider again your list of community assets. Which of these assets, if destroyed or seriously damaged, would produce a catastrophic result?

Would the destruction of any one asset result in catastrophe?

Would the destruction of some collection of assets produce a catastrophe?

If you can envision a catastrophic result, is it because of the asset not being available or is it because of the public's reaction to the asset not being available?

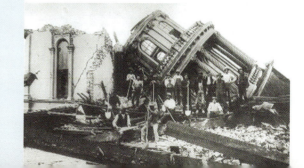

Santa Rosa City Hall, 1906.
Source: The Steinbrugge Collection of the UC Berkeley Earthquake Engineering Research Center

CHAPTER 2 — RECOGNIZE THREATS

Community Assets	Most Direct Catastrophe	Largest Sense of Catastrophe	Most Immediate Disruption	Most Long-Term Disruption
water supply				
food supply				
waste and sanitation services				
sewage treatment				
public health				
primary health care				
emergency health care				
long-term and geriatric health care				
housing supply				
electricity supply				
natural gas supply				
gasoline supply				
continuity of government				
police services				
public works services				
fire services				
judicial services				
taxation and public revenue				
rail transportation system				
road transportation system				
air transportation system				
water transportation system				
telephone communications				
radio broadcasting				
television broadcasting				
Internet				
commercial (wholesale and retail) sector				
manufacturing sector				
financial services sector				
professional services sector				
distribution sector				
hospitality sector				
public schools				
colleges and universities				
sports events				
religious events				
cultural events				
political events				

There are **several variables** at play that can determine whether or not an event is catastrophic or is perceived as catastrophic.

The **scope** and **scale** of death and destruction is a major factor. The **effectiveness of the immediate response** is another. The **speed of recovery efforts** is very important. Whether or not the public is **surprised** or **has been prepared** for the attack and its consequences can be crucial. All of these factors influence public perception of the event and determine whether its consequences, in the words of Richard Posner, "produce a harm so great and sudden as to seem discontinuous with the flow of events that preceded it."

Read the list of community assets at left. Is unavailability of any of these community assets for a period of three days likely to produce a catastrophe? What about one week or one month? Where would unavailability cause the most immediate death and destruction? Where would unavailability cause the most long-term disruption?

Is the **public's response** to the unavailability of any of these assets likely to produce a sense of catastrophe even if response and recovery is reasonably effective? Is the public response to unavailability due to a natural threat likely to be different than if the cause is accidental or intentional?

We might say that catastrophe is in the eye of the beholder. The same consequence can mean something very different to various audiences depending on their attitudes and proximity to the consequence. Something that is entirely catastrophic at the local level may not have catastrophic implications for others elsewhere.

Local officials are clearly the most motivated to prevent and mitigate a local catastrophe.

FEAR AS A THREAT AMPLIFIER

In the aftermath of 9/11 many anticipated follow-on attacks. Based on this expectation travel—especially air travel—fell precipitously. The reduction in travel had a significant impact on restaurants, hotels, and related industries.

The World Trade Center towers were just a few blocks from the New York Stock Exchange. WTC had housed several large financial services firms. The Exchange was closed for a week. After it reopened the Dow Jones Industrial Average fell over 14 percent in only four days.

Surveys of New Yorkers three to six months after the 9/11 attacks found that over half self-reported emotional complications which were perceived to be related to the attacks. (DeLisi, Maurizio, et al)

Panic is almost never the problem. Time after time the immediate response of the public to most disasters is controlled, contained, and even courageous. But fear does play a role, especially in the days and weeks following a disaster.

In the immediate aftermath of 9/11 it was often said, "this changes everything." This is how a catastrophe is perceived. **Catastrophe is the psychological and social response to a disastrous event**, as much as the physical result itself.

Identifying fear as a threat and working to eliminate or reduce this threat is an important part of preventing catastrophe.

Fear is the result of imagination as much as direct involvement. In the aftermath of a 1995 poison gas attack on the Tokyo subway the "worried-well" challenged the healthcare system much more than the actual victims of the attack.

To prepare the public's imagination, try to TALK before, during, and after the event.

TALK consists of four methods:

Threats Identified—Identify specific threats in advance of an event. There is almost no empirical evidence to support the concern that such discussion increases public anxiety. Rather, the more specific information that is provided on a potential threat the more the public expresses confidence and avoids fear.

Assurance Communicated—Be realistic and specific regarding meaningful preparations. The public will be assured if they have evidence authorities are aware of the threat, are taking reasonable actions to reduce or respond to the threat, and are being proactive not just reactive.

Leadership Exercised—The very public involvement of senior leaders, both elected and appointed, is a crucial aspect of fear management. This is helpful in advance of a threat. It is fundamental to an effective response to an actual threat. Modeling calm, thoughtful and courageous behavior encourages similar behavior in others.

Knowledge Distributed—The more information that is available regarding both potential threats and response to threats, the less likely fear will overwhelm the public's imagination.

The news media is an essential component in any effective approach to managing fear. Informing the media in advance, involving the media in catastrophe training and exercising, and establishing effective relationships with the media in advance of a catastrophe is one of the best investments to avoid catastrophe.

Two articles on media relations are available on the CD: *Leadership through Media* by Elizabeth L. Robbins and *The Role of Broadcast Media in Homeland Security Communication* by Frank Sesno.

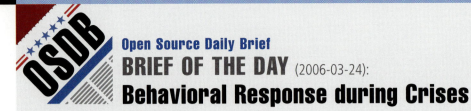

Open Source Daily Brief
BRIEF OF THE DAY (2006-03-24): Behavioral Response during Crises

The psychological impacts, effects, and consequences of traumatic events are important components of terrorism prevention and planning. Terrorists attack in order to evoke feelings of fear, helplessness, vulnerability, and grief. Communication during the midst of crisis influences individual behavioral responses to disaster. Emergency responders need to understand and anticipate behavioral responses of victims of crises as well as individuals close to the victims.

Paul DeVito, Ph.D., Director of the Early Responder's Distance Learning Center at Saint Joseph's University, Philadelphia, suggests "emergency responders should be confident, flexible, empathetic and team players who can take decisive actions while maintaining a hopeful outlook." He cites Rudy Giuliani's response to the September 11, 2001 attacks as an example of how to accomplish empathy and optimism during a crisis. In response to Giuliani being asked "[h]ow many people were killed?" Giuliani responded, "I think the number is greater than we can bear." DeVito highlights, "Giuliani acknowledged the enormity of the tragedy, extended his sympathies, and reassured people that everyone involved in the relief and recovery effort would do everything they could to make things better."

Emergency responders are encouraged to project a sense of control over crises and to reduce panic and fear by providing good information. The treatment of terrorism victims immediately after a terror event directly affects their recovery from the event. A recent article by Mark A. Stebnicki, Associate Professor at East Carolina University, School of Allied Health Sciences, recognizes two types of survivors: primary survivors and secondary survivors. Stebnicki defines primary survivors as persons "who have personally witnessed or have been survivors of stressful and traumatic events." Secondary survivors are those individuals who are "exposed by learning of the event through relatives, friends, acquaintances, or exposure to repeated accounts by the media." However, Stebnicki acknowledges, "many persons may experience secondary traumatic stress which may be as real as those persons considered to be primary survivors." Thus, highly skilled and empathetic communication by emergency responders can reduce the trauma of survivors.

Situations where responders also become primary survivors/victims, as with Hurricane Katrina in 2005, are particularly difficult. "This is unprecedented in our country," said Dr. Howard Osofsky, chairman of psychiatry at the LSU Medical School Health Sciences Department. "There is no disaster that has had the amount of trauma for a department that this has, where so many police officers have lost homes, been separated from their families, had loved ones living in other places with no idea when they'll return." In a tribute to their oath, courage and dedication, the majority of New Orleans Police Officers ignored their personal problems, according to police spokesperson Marlon Defillo, "[w]e have approximately 1,450 commissioned persons who are working under some very adverse conditions. It's a tribute to those officers who are working very hard to do the right thing."

PREVENTION RELEVANCE: The better first responders understand their own behavior and the behavior of victims during times of crisis and uncertainty, the greater their ability to reduce the social and psychological damage done.

PREVENTION TECHNIQUES: Training emergency responders to understand and empathize with primary and secondary survivors enables them to affect victims of terrorism positively.

PREVENTION THOUGHT: Information Sharing Do any obstacles currently keep emergency responders from seeking training regarding behavioral impacts of trauma? What types of training do you think would prove most useful?

The Open Source Daily Brief is a service of the Institute for Preventive Strategies (©IPS). You can register to receive the OSDBs at www.preventivestrategies.net.

RECOGNIZE THREATS:
Chapter Review

What are the most serious threats facing your community? Which of these threats are potentially catastrophic?

Are there specific terrorist groups active in your community? If so, what are their intentions: Nationalist, ideological, religious, or other?

Given their intentions, which group or groups might consider causing a catastrophe?

Of those who might want to cause a catastrophe, do they have a known capability for causing catastrophe? A potential capability?

Even if there are no such groups present in your community, outside groups—domestic or international—might choose your community as a target. Is your community especially vulnerable to any particular weapon of catastrophe?

Most terrorist groups tend to "live off the land." They access local resources to develop a weapon's capability. The principal categories of catastrophic weapons include toxins, chemicals, biological agents, radiological materials, and nuclear devices. Which of these weapons resources are locally available? Is your local community especially vulnerable to any of these weapons?

What are your community's most serious natural and accidental threats?

Do you have a local history of natural or accidental disasters? If so, is there a pattern that should influence your preparedness?

What are your community's most critical assets?

Which assets are most important to your community's survival and recovery?

Which assets deserve the most protection?

What is the best process for selecting these critical assets?

Whether an event is catastrophic or not depends greatly on how the public interprets the event. What can be done before, during, and after the execution of an intentional threat to manage public readiness and response?

APPLY WHAT YOU HAVE LEARNED

Use your CD to access the Threat Recognition Advanced Exercise. Select the **Chapter 2** Certificate Course link located in the Online Exercises section of your CD.

It is now 9 months before a planned terrorist attack. The threat is organizing, planning and becoming real. Can you identify the most probable targets and their vulnerabilities based on the perceived threat? **You are collaborating and sharing information to identify threats in the fictional jurisdiction of San Luis Rey®.** Your efforts to collaborate and share information are paying off. You are receiving information from your collaboration partners. But, even with this information, you must make threat and vulnerability choices.

- Will your choices reduce the risk of an intentional incident from occurring?
- Have you accurately identified threat capabilities?
- Do you have enough information?
- Is your collaboration network sufficient?

See how your choices compare to peers'. The clock is ticking.

Note: If you have already enrolled in the Homeland Security Terrorism Prevention Certificate Course for Fire Service Professionals (©IPS) you can go directly to the exercise by using the Online Exercises Direct Access links on your CD or by typing this URL into your browser's address window:

www.preventivestrategies.net/go/mhfs-adv-ex-threats

For first time access, use this initial URL:
www.preventivestrategies.net/go/mhfs-enroll

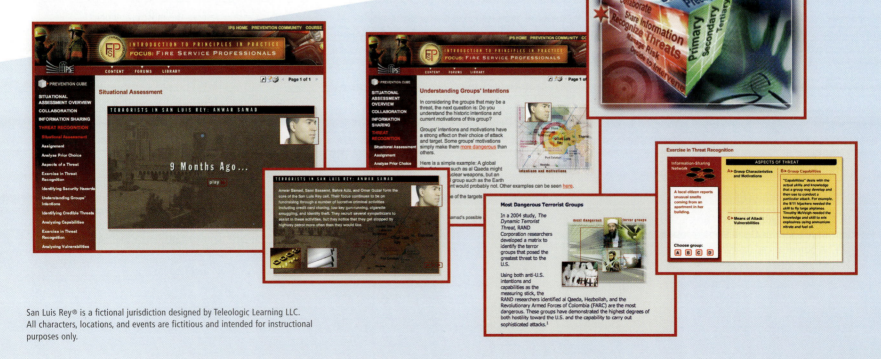

San Luis Rey® is a fictional jurisdiction designed by Teleologic Learning LLC. All characters, locations, and events are fictitious and intended for instructional purposes only.

CHAPTER 3 — SHARE INFORMATION

Share Information

✓ *In this chapter you will learn:*
- **How to organize an effective strategic intelligence function.**
- **How to choose appropriate intelligence targets.**
- **How to access and gather Open Source information.**
- **How to analyze Open Source information.**
- **How to develop helpful intelligence products.**
- **How to consume intelligence products.**

Were you able to answer with accuracy and confidence most of the questions posed in the previous chapter on Recognizing Threats? If so, you are unusually well informed. It is possible to imagine many natural, accidental, and intentional threats. To accurately identify which threats should receive your ongoing attention requires significant information and analysis.

To prevent or mitigate catastrophe requires making tough choices about threats and application of resources to those threats. **The more information—and the better information—available, the more likely your community can make good choices.**

Better information is the result of gathering, sifting, comparing, confirming, and considering information in order to apply accurate information to a well-defined problem. We are all drowning in information. Finding the right information and focusing it on a recognized problem means to transform raw information into actionable intelligence.

Spy novels, movies, and television shows give us the impression that the intelligence business is an action packed infiltration of the enemy's inner circles or super-sophisticated satellite reconnaissance. Most of the intelligence business actually involves looking carefully at information that is available to everyone. You probably don't have access to classified information, but that doesn't mean you can't contribute to the overall intelligence process or benefit from it. Some have estimated that over 90 percent of intelligence reported in the Presidential Daily Brief—a highly classified CIA intelligence product—is drawn from open sources.

Every community needs a good intelligence function that draws upon the insights, observations, and expertise of all first responder agencies. As a Department of Justice White Paper recently commented: "… intelligence tells officials everything they need to know before they knowledgeably choose a course

Most of the intelligence business actually involves looking carefully at information that is available to everyone.

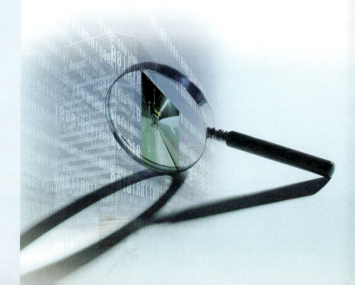

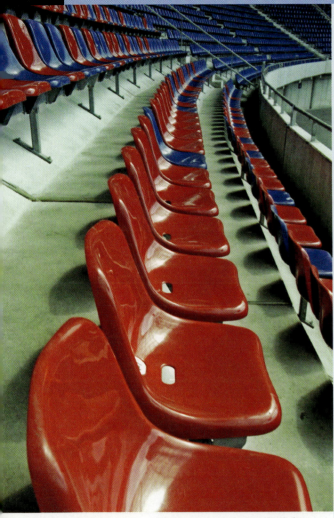

Source: iStockphoto

Identify, assess, and prioritize potential sites in your community with vulnerabilities that serve as "force multipliers."

of action." (*Intelligence-Led Policing: The New Intelligence Architecture*). The fire service can contribute to that overall effort and help ensure a fully all-hazards awareness of risk.

Knowledgeable choices are better choices.

STRATEGIC INTELLIGENCE AND FIRE INTELLIGENCE

To prevent rather than respond, you need an accurate understanding of natural, accidental, and intentional threats. Decision-makers need strategic information to establish priorities, make plans, allocate resources, develop training, and coordinate across agencies and governments. Yet, strategic information originates from many sources in the community, including observations made in the course of routine fire service practices. Strategic information aims to inform strategic choices. Strategic choices are those that enhance the readiness of a community long before catastrophe is at hand.

Fire information developed from tactical activities can inform intelligence efforts relevant to homeland security. Fire intelligence has been defined as: "Information derived by the fire service for the fire service, and for the utilization of others, intended to provide meaningful and trustworthy direction and support to decision makers in pursuit of the homeland security mission" (Flynn, John).

The location of sprinklers in a high-rise structure is information collected by a fire department to understand the fire suppression system of the structure. The location of exits from that same building is information collected by a building or other appropriate municipal department. Combining those two pieces of information provides fire intelligence. Including such fire intelligence into threat and vulnerability assessments for that same high-rise structure adds to strategic intelligence.

Strategy is proactive rather than responsive.

Strategic needs differ considerably from **tactical needs**. **Strategic intelligence is much more concerned with how and why, rather than who and what.** Because strategic intelligence is more interested in how and why, rather than who or what, it does not focus nearly so much on suspected terrorists and/or organizations. Strategic intelligence—especially in regards to preventing catastrophe—is much more concerned about **assessing the capability of a potential threat regardless of the source**.

Capability Based Assessment emerged from post-Cold War efforts within the Department of Defense to plan for future threats. Instead of focusing on a specific enemy, such as the Soviet Union or Al-Qaeda, place attention on anticipating different kinds of threats regardless of the specific source. In other words, try to detect potentially harmful activities or resources in the community that can multiply the effects of a disaster. Then, apply public safety resources to: 1) deter the potential activity by depriving terrorists access to the capability, or 2) diminish the impact from natural or accidental disasters (Martinez). This approach is especially appropriate for prevention of catastrophe. Many recognize the approach as a fire service best practice.

The first line of strategic intelligence gathering involves identifying, assessing, and prioritizing potential sites in your community with vulnerabilities that serve as "force multipliers" for natural, accidental, or intentional catastrophes. Of specific interest are those sites with potential value for terrorists to strike due to their "force-multiplier" potential. Sites with "force-multiplier" potential not only increase the harm from intentional threats but also from natural and accidental threats.

Information about vulnerabilities in your community is available from a variety of sources including the Risk Management Program (Section 112 r of the Clean Air Act) and your Local Emergency Planning Committee (LEPC). The Environmental Protection Agency supports compliance with the Emergency Planning and Community Right-to-Know Act (EPCRA) under Title III of the Superfund Amendments and Reauthorization Act of 1986. The EPCRA provides the legal basis for a "firefighter right-to-know" about hazardous materials stored or processed by industry in communities, and the states have passed enabling legislation to support compliance with the federal statute (Hawkins).

The LEPC database is available online. (See the link on the CD.) It provides a search capability to display information about 3000 listings across the United States. As the U.S. Environmental Protection Agency website indicates, "Local Emergency Planning Committees (LEPCs) provide a forum for emergency management agencies, responders, industry and the public to work together to understand chemical hazards in the community, develop emergency plans in case of an accidental release, and always look for ways to prevent chemical accidents. Local industries must provide information to LEPCs about chemical hazards. LEPCs are required by law to make this information available to any citizen who requests it. You can make a difference by attending an LEPC meeting or joining your LEPC." ("Chemicals in Your Community…")

If you are unable to obtain information from your community's LEPC, or the LEPC database, on what kinds of materials industrial facilities in your area use and store, ask your fire company officers to **consider doing a**

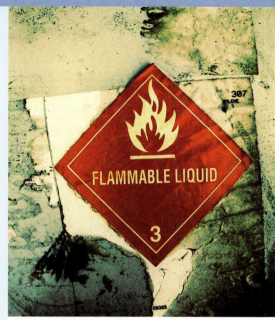

Source: iStockphoto

Force Multiplier is a term that originated in the military. According to the Department of Defense it is **"a capability that, when added to and employed by a combat force, significantly increases the combat potential of that force."** The interaction of a natural threat, such as a flood, with an infrastructure vulnerability, such as spillage from a refinery, multiplies the force or impact of the original threat.

CHAPTER 3 — SHARE INFORMATION

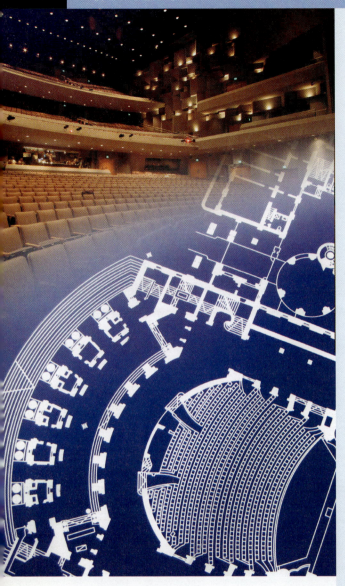

Routine prevention activities such as pre-incident inspections offer intelligence gathering opportunities.

pre-incident inspection. As part of a visit to a facility, you can learn a great deal by making the following inquiries to management:

1. Ask what types of processing occur at the facility as well as what is stored there and how much.
2. Ask what types of chemicals the facility uses, stores, or manufactures, and request the material safety data sheets (MSDSs) for them.
3. Ask about potential environmental impacts from leaks, fires, or spills.
4. Ask about community impacts from leaks, fires, or spills.
5. Ask whether planning for a worst-case event needs to include evacuation of the local area.
6. Ask about the extent of commercial impact from a worst-case event.

(Shelley and Cole)

Even though the EPCRA legislation provides wide-ranging authority for the fire service to gather information about hazardous materials stored or processed at local facilities, it does not cover all circumstances.

The October 5, 2006 fire at EQ Industrial Services, a hazmat transfer facility in Apex, North Carolina, exemplifies both the opportunities and constraints in taking a proactive approach to information gathering on industrial facilities. The Apex fire demonstrated the importance to fire service personnel of knowing what hazardous materials are stored in facilities in their community. It also demonstrated the practical limitations of the EPCRA in supporting the firefighter right-to-know authority. The Fire Chief of the Apex Fire Department, Mark Haraway, had attempted to identify the hazardous materials handled at EQ Industrial Services in advance. However, the quantities of those materials fell below thresholds defined by the EPCRA reporting requirements. In addition, the site's inventory changed regularly, meaning that the facility was only required to maintain a daily manifest (White).

The inability to develop accurate information about the chemicals stored at EQ resulted in firefighters necessarily presuming the worst-case on the night of the explosion at the facility, leading to an evacuation of the entire 17,000 residents of the town. After arriving on the scene, the representative of EQ could only describe the contents of the warehouse in generalities (Coleman, "Apex Wants Full Hazmat Disclosure").

The North Carolina Chemical Safety Board indicated that the fire raged out of control only after it spread from an area where waste pool chemicals, cyanide sludge and other materials were stored. The facility design emphasized preventing spills but not maximizing fire suppression. For instance, a simple 6-inch curb at the warehouse separated oxides from flammable wastes ("Apex Facility Fire Prevention Shortcomings").

In June 2007, the U.S. Chemical Safety Board announced its finding that, even though the cause of the fire remains unidentified, its intensity resulted from the presence of improperly handled, unspent oxygen generators. Commercial aircraft use the generators to provide supplemental oxygen in drop-down masks when the cabin depressurizes. Without the oxygen to feed the flames provided by the unspent generators, the fire would have died out quickly or burned so slowly that firefighters would have had little trouble extinguishing it. An aircraft maintenance shop transferred the oxygen generators to the EQ facility without expending the devices (Hartsoe).

As a result of the Apex fire, North Carolina imposed new regulations stipulating that, among other requirements, companies applying for a hazardous waste permit must take certain proactive steps relative to the surrounding community and emergency agencies. Those steps include
- notifying businesses and residents within a quarter mile and periodically sending out information about the company's emergency response plan;
- providing local governments and emergency personnel with information about what is stored and contingency plans for emergencies; and
- maintaining a list of chemicals stored in an off site location.

(Bonner)

Whether an earthquake, operating error, or terrorist action takes down your community's electrical grid is less important than the fact that the power is out. The capability to shut down electricity across a broad area is characteristic of many natural, accidental, and intentional threats. Biological hazards come in natural (pandemic), accidental (toxic spills), and intentional (anthrax, smallpox, etc.) forms. It is the capability for biological harm that may provide the best strategic information for decision-makers.

Catastrophe is often the result of force multiplication: where a natural, accidental or intentional threat interacts with existing vulnerabilities or another threat. **The fire service is uniquely qualified to gather information, analyze, and understand the vulnerabilities and threat capabilities that exist in a community.** Working with other preparedness professions the fire service can apply this understanding to reduce the risk of catastrophe.

At the strategic level, the focus on capabilities as opposed to specific actors avoids many of the civil liberties issues involved in collecting information on specific individuals and organizations. In some cases, the strategic process may expose information that raises the issue of "reasonable suspicion," but at that point the purpose of the intelligence moves from the strategic to the tactical, meaning the fire service shares the information with appropriate law enforce-

Strategic Intelligence— assessing threat **capabilities**

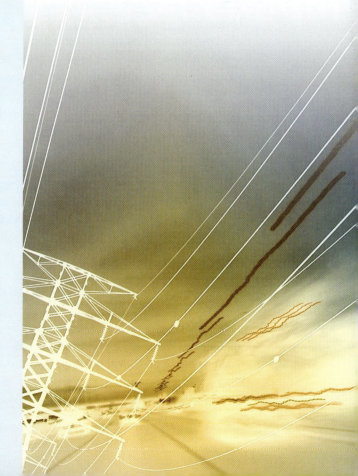

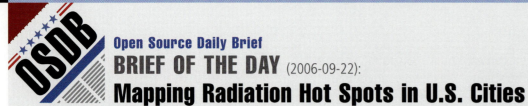

Open Source Daily Brief
BRIEF OF THE DAY (2006-09-22):
Mapping Radiation Hot Spots in U.S. Cities

Concerns about the potential damage from terrorists using weapons of mass destruction have increased dramatically after the September 11, 2001 attacks. Authorities focus attention on the threat of nuclear weapons, but also increasingly focus on the threat of terrorists deploying "dirty bombs." A dirty bomb threatens to spread contaminants across an area, killing people and destroying physical structures with a conventional blast, while leaving it virtually useless because of radiation. There are differing views on the effectiveness of a dirty bomb in spreading large-scale contamination. Yet, concern about the threat of such devices is serious enough that over 10,000 portable radiation detectors are now in use by state, local, and federal homeland security efforts.

A recent Government Accountability Office (GAO) report indicated that the Department of Energy used its Remote Sensing capability to conduct aerial background radiation surveys in New York City last summer at the request of the New York City Police Department. New York is the only city in the United States to request such a survey so far. The survey located 80 hot spots of radiation in the city, ranging from medical facilities to naturally occurring sources. It also identified an area of Gateway National Park in Staten Island as emitting dangerously high levels of radium. The area was about the size of a football field. The NYPD has since fenced off the area.

The GAO report criticized the Department of Energy (DOE) and Homeland Security (DHS) for failing to encourage other cities at risk of terror attacks to request such aerial surveys. The Domestic Nuclear Detection Office (DNDO) of DHS is "responsible for developing, testing, and deploying radiation detection equipment to detect and prevent the smuggling of nuclear and radiological materials at U.S. points of entry, such as seaports and border crossings." DNDO also helps state and local governments in detecting and identifying illicit nuclear and radiological materials. However, if DHS fails to prevent smuggling of nuclear or radiological materials into the United States, DOE must search for and locate the materials, and measure contamination levels. The GAO report notes that, without baseline data from the aerial background radiation surveys, measuring contamination levels after a dirty bomb attack becomes much more difficult.

It summarized the benefits of such surveys as follows: "There are significant benefits to conducting aerial background radiation surveys of U.S. cities. Specifically, the surveys can be used to compare changes in radiation levels to (1) help detect radiological threats in U.S. cities more quickly and (2) measure contamination levels after a radiological attack to assist in and reduce the costs of cleanup efforts. Despite the benefits, only one major city has been surveyed. Neither DOE nor DHS has mission responsibility for conducting these surveys, and there are no plans to conduct additional surveys."

GAO indicated that the absence of baseline information from such surveys could cause law enforcement to lose valuable time investigating sources of radiation that existed before an attack and pose no threat. Moreover, without baseline information on radiation hot spots, the time and cost of cleanup after an attack with a dirty bomb are likely to increase significantly.

PREVENTION RELEVANCE: The threat that terrorists could smuggle a nuclear weapon into the United States, or smuggle radioactive materials to use in a dirty bomb, is a worst-case scenario for a terrorist attack.

PREVENTION TECHNIQUES: Map radioactive hot spots in major cities in the United States to establish a benchmark for use in response efforts in the event of a "dirty bomb" attack.

PREVENTION THOUGHT: Risk Management
Do you think it makes sense for all the major urban areas in the United States to request an aerial survey of radiation hot spots from the Department of Energy?

The Open Source Daily Brief is a service of the Institute for Preventive Strategies (©IPS). You can register to receive the OSDBs at www.preventivestrategies.net.

CHAPTER 3 — SHARE INFORMATION

ment agencies for additional, tactical intelligence gathering.

The collecting, analyzing and sharing of well-chosen information is important in making wise strategic choices. The purpose of strategic intelligence and information sharing is to defend the lives and liberties of your neighbors. Doing the work in a manner that does not threaten those liberties is also important.

More consideration is given to this issue in two readings on your CD: *Thinking about Civil Liberty and Terrorism* by Paul Rosenzweig and *Principled Prudence: Civil Liberties and the Homeland Security Practitioner* by Laura W. Murphy.

*Being **strategic** is to be explicit and purposeful about how various forces that influence your **context** can be effectively engaged to help in achieving an important goal.*

A strategist seeks to command the context.

THE INTELLIGENCE PROCESS

The intelligence process occurs in different ways depending on purposes and organizations. The intelligence you gather to pre-plan for natural or accidental catastrophe differs from that gathered for intentional catastrophe only to the extent that the latter can involve observations emerging from a routine activity, such as an inspection, or a non-routine activity such as a fire. Those observations typically involve objects or activities that are suspicious in a particular context.

Some jurisdictions are capable of putting in place specific counterterrorism units within their fire departments. Cities such as New York, Philadelphia, and Los Angeles are a few examples. Los Angeles, for instance, began collaborating in the counterterrorism efforts of the region in 1998 as a part of the Los Angeles Terrorism Early Warning (TEW) Group. The Los Angeles Fire Department (LAFD) organized a Terrorism Liaison Officer (TLO) Program in 2005 to facilitate information sharing with internal and external partners in the urban area. The TLO essentially serves as a local point of contact (POC) for the Joint Terrorism Task Force (JTTF). However, LAFD participation in the counter-terrorism effort more recently resulted in a Special Operations Division with a distinct organiza-

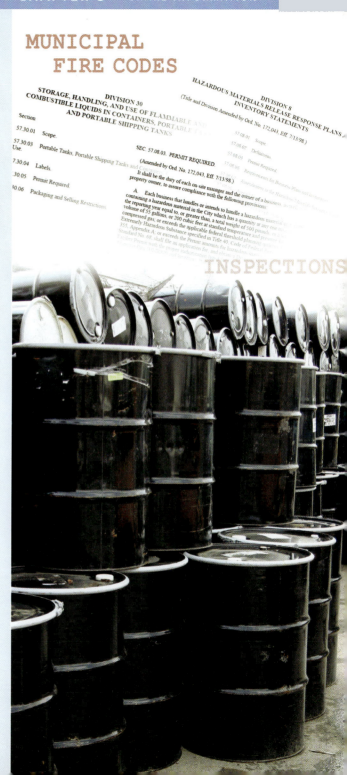

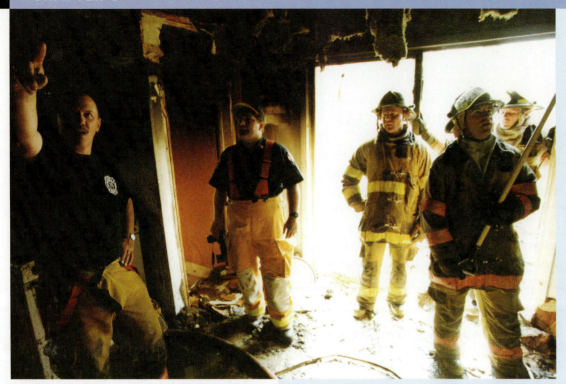

Fire investigation
Source: Bloomington Fire Department, Bloomington, IL

The process of collecting and analyzing information draws from and extends traditional activities of the fire service.

tional structure within LAFD, including a Division Commander, three Battalion Chiefs, and numerous Captains in specialized units. The TLO program in particular provides an information channel for firefighters to refer observations of suspicious conduct to the JTTF for investigation. On the other hand, TLO members assigned to the TEW are able to report any information gained through their analysis to field personnel who can adjust operational procedures accordingly (Welch).

The FDNY organizes its intelligence sharing primarily through the Center for Terrorism and Disaster Preparedness (CTDP) and the Bureau of Fire Investigation. Members of the FDNY Bureau of Fire Investigation serve on the JTTF. The FDNY also began direct information sharing with the DHS Office of Intelligence and Analysis in 2007. Additionally, FDNY's Risk Assessment and Target Hazard (RATH) program coordinates site evaluations to identify site vulnerability and consequence management issues (New York City Fire Department, "Written Statement of the FDNY…"; New York City Fire Department, "Terrorism and Disaster Preparedness Strategy…"). Institutional changes, like those in the LAFD and FDNY, are an important part of fire service efforts to incorporate prevention and preparedness into strategy and tactics, especially for the counterterrorism mission.

Creating new institutional roles is not in itself sufficient to meet the challenges faced. Incorporating a focus on preventing terrorism into the routine activities of line personnel means educating all fire service professionals on how to recognize relevant information and what to do with it. For example, in his survey research of 529 fire service personnel in the FDNY, John Flynn found several limitations in the department's current management practices for terrorism information. Seventy-two percent of respondents reported that FDNY has encouraged them to observe, identify, or report indications of terrorist activity. Yet, "only 15% of respondents reported being aware of an entity within the department that is specifically designated to obtain terrorist related information and distribute it for response support purposes [In addition,] 92.2% of respondents are unaware of an organized structure for the transfer of terrorism information from other entities (such as the NYPD and FBI) to the FDNY" ("Terrorism Information Management within the New York City Fire Department…").

Regardless of a fire department's ability to dedicate staff to the counterterrorism effort, the process of collecting information and analyzing it draws from and extends traditional activities of the fire service. "Pre-incident" inspections of occupancies with a potential for high hazard, i.e. high rises, industrial facilities, etc. are a part of many fire departments' routine activities. Indeed, the hazardous materials monitoring equipment carried by most fire department units can detect radiation and identify materials useful in making dirty bombs. In addition, identifying unusual symptoms in medical patients can alert EMS personnel to the presence of a bioterrorist or pandemic threat ("Terrorism and Disaster Preparedness Strategy…").

Training all firefighters to recognize "force multipliers" and associated cascading failure potential in a natural or accidental catastrophe, as well as indicators of potential terrorist planning, is a part of the intelligence process for preparation and prevention (Welch). The important point to take away from the survey research on FDNY reported above is that recognizing suspicious or threatening capabilities is only part of the challenge facing the fire service in preventing catastrophe. Each fire department needs to make sure fire service personnel know who to share such information with.

Five-Steps

Information is processed to become intelligence. Some say, "Intelligence is information plus analysis." Yet, analysis is only one element in the overall process. Following is a **five-step description:**

1. Choose Pre-Incident Intelligence Targets: What do you need to know about facilities in your community and how will you use the knowledge? Given those purposes, what are the most promising sources of accurate information? Given your available resources, which intelligence targets are must-have? Which are nice-to-have? Targets could range from bulk explosives trucks servicing quarries just outside your community, to mapping out primary and secondary water supplies for fire suppression in the community, or regularly scheduled shipments of hazardous materials moving through your community by rail or truck. You want to choose pre-incident targets for developing intelligence based on vulnerability and threat assessments (Bachman, "Preincident Intelligence of Quarries"; Bachman, "Water Supply Preincident Intelligence"; Deonarine, "Industrial Terrorism").

What do you need to know about facilities in your community?

Intelligence targets could include shipments moving through your community by rail or truck.

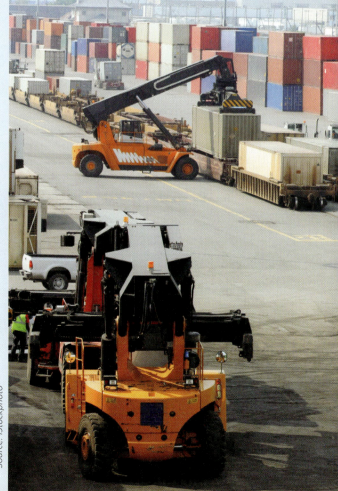

Source: iStockphoto

CHAPTER 3 — SHARE INFORMATION

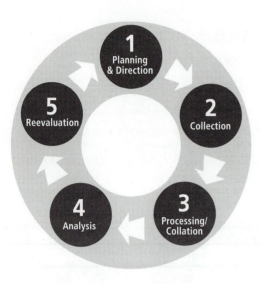

The version of the Intelligence Process shown above is from *Intelligence-Led Policing: The New Intelligence Architecture*.

2. **Collect Data and Information:** Consistent with your targets and your resources, what do you gather? What do you ask? Scan broadly. Develop a personal network of trusted sources. Gather both explicit and implicit information. Dig deep when you can. Look for interrelationships.

3. **Organize and Analyze Information:** Are there strategic and operational assumptions that should be tested? Can you confirm or refute these assumptions? Compare your information. Look for patterns. Look for aberrations in the patterns. Apply the scientific method to your information.

4. **Produce Intelligence Products:** Who are the principal decision-makers related to preventing catastrophe? How do they make decisions? What is their preferred means of receiving and processing information? Create intelligence products that match the needs of your consumers.

5. **Consume Intelligence Products:** Who are your consumers? Are there different levels of consumers? Do your consumers understand how to use your products? How can you better prepare the consumers to understand and use what you are producing?

In the case of natural and accidental catastrophes, your intelligence function is not concerned with secrecy. Instead, you are trying to find and highlight critical information that often goes unnoticed. You are trying to see

How is the model depicted above different from the five-step process shown at right?

_____
_____
_____
_____
_____
_____
_____

C-COP-C
A Five Step Intelligence Process

- **Consume** intelligence products.
- **Produce** intelligence products.
- **Organize** and **analyze** data and information.
- **Collect** data and information.
- **Choose** intelligence targets.

the tree in the midst of the forest.

The same is mostly true regarding the threat of intentional catastrophe. Terrorists certainly try to keep secrets. Yet, just as fire behavior is observable, so are terrorism planning actions and behaviors. "Firefighters train to recognize certain conditions that warn of backdraft, flashover, or rollover…We can reduce the danger of terrorism through education and training" (Welch). For example, in reconnaissance, logistics, ordinance, and other operations terrorists engage in observable behavior that fire service professionals can learn to recognize. Therefore, as fire service personnel go about routines like inspections and responding to alarms, they can add any suspicious situations to their typical observations about fire extinguishers, blocked exits, etc. Terrorists must make and test weapons, "or components of weapons systems before they are deployed. The potential for fire personnel to respond to a test gone wrong or preoperational test is considerable" (Martinez and McLoughlin). On the other hand, intelligence received from others in your collaboration network, such as the local point of contact (POC) with the FBI's Joint Terrorism Task Force (JTTF) or the U.S. Attorney's Anti-Terrorism Advisory Council (ATAC), can inform actions taken to counter a potential attack. The actions are sometimes as simple as securing facilities to limit access, doing high-profile inspections, or developing teams specializing in rapid response against specific threats.

On television, the drama of counterterrorism usually involves penetrating a local terrorist cell. Such clandestine activity is the exception. Rather, **developing a situational awareness to help you and others keep focused on potential threats** is the most likely strategy for successful prevention of catastrophe in your community. Many believe a border agent who was sufficiently aware of context noticed subtly strange behavior and thwarted an attack on Seattle by a ferry passenger referred to as the "Millennium bomber," named Ahmed Ressam. As Brett Martinez, a fire marshal for the Suffolk County (NY) Fire Rescue and Emergency Services puts it, "The concepts of counterterrorism operation for the fire service are not complicated or dangerous; they simply

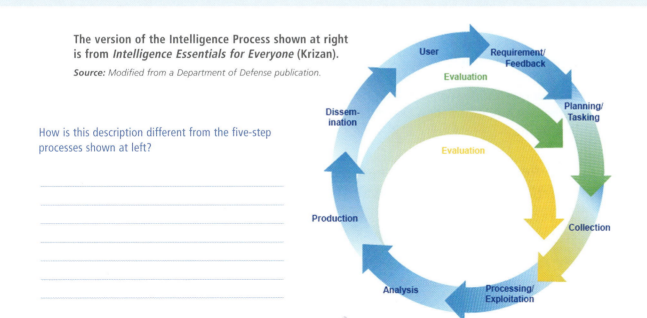

The version of the Intelligence Process shown at right is from *Intelligence Essentials for Everyone* (Krizan).

Source: Modified from a Department of Defense publication.

How is this description different from the five-step processes shown at left?

Something is **implicit** when it is implied but not directly expressed.

Implicit knowledge is sometimes intuitive knowledge, an expert guess, or a professional's experienced judgment.

How you organize your resources to achieve purpose is a fundamental choice. In your opinion what would be a good purpose for your community's **strategic** intelligence function?

___

Will your fire service organization invest any time, any money, any personnel?

___

involve doing the same things we do every day. The only difference is that now it has become necessary for us to stay informed, be alert to everything we can, and pass any concerns or information gained onto the proper agencies" ("The Fire Service and Counterterrorism…").

Are firefighters in your department trained to recognize suspicious situations? Considering Martinez's point, if firefighters from your department notice 50 gallons of chlorine in a basement for a house without a swimming pool, do they know what to do? If, while doing a smoke detector installation, they notice multiple passports on a kitchen table all with the same picture on them, would they consider passing along that information? On the other hand, would they consider the observations irrelevant to their task and forget about them at the end of the response or shift? Would they simply think to themselves that it is the cops' job?

We survive information overload by screening out information that seems irrelevant.

An effective strategic intelligence function highlights the relevance of factors that will enable us to prevent or mitigate catastrophe.

CHOOSE INTELLIGENCE TARGETS

There are many needs for good intelligence. The goal of prevention is significantly different from fire investigation. Prevention benefits from situational awareness before an event. A fire investigation is usually focused on a specific question after an event, asking what caused it and whether the causes were accident or intentional. A fire investigation also involves analysis of data to determine where fires occur, under what conditions, and whether they follow specific patterns. An analysis of fire patterns can, for example, uncover evidence of arson.

Thinking in similar terms about terrorism can also make patterns visible, reflecting the routine activities of the target. For example, terrorist attacks against financial institutions tend to occur between 0800 and 1000 hours, Monday through Friday. Attack sites are characteristically on or near mass transit hubs. On the other hand, terrorist attacks on resort or vacation sites typically occur between 1900 and 0000 hours, most often on Thursday, Friday, or Saturday nights. Attack sites are usually nightclubs, restaurants, or other venues where large numbers of people congregate (Martinez and McLoughlin).

The strategic intelligence needed to prevent catastrophe is often available openly and usually benefits from a broad sharing of both information and analysis.

Your resources are always limited. Time, money, and personnel are often constant. How you organize your resources—to do what—is a fundamental choice. What priority will your community give to preventing catastrophe?

Judge Richard Posner has written, "We have seen that the levels of current expenditures to combat the major catastrophic risks… assume the risks are much smaller than they probably are. We have also seen that there are many possibilities… for responding to the catastrophic risks without breaking the bank. Were the dangers posed by the catastrophic risks and the opportunities for minimizing those risks more generally recognized, the United States and the world would rouse themselves to effective action, and the world would be a safer place." (*Catastrophe: Risk and Response*)

Catastrophic threats are natural, accidental, and intentional. What do you need—what do your consumers of intelligence products need—to know about each of these threats?

Natural threats are probably the easiest to monitor. Weather events are only a computer-click or remote button away. Geologic events are more difficult to predict, but plenty of resources are available. The CD includes links to National Earthquake Information Center and others. Check the threat of earthquake for your region or community. You might be surprised. Major media is extensively covering the threat of Pandemic Influenza.

More specific surveillance information is available from the Centers for Disease Control and Prevention at www.pandemicflu.gov.

In your local community **the emergency management agency, public health agency and other preparedness professionals may already be expert in gathering and analyzing information on natural threats.** You will probably find it helpful to develop relationships with these offices.

The strategic intelligence function can help decision-makers recognize natural threats—and especially the threat of natural catastrophe—as something for which they need to plan, train, and exercise. A hurricane, earthquake, pandemic, or other big-footprint disaster will seriously stress any fire service agency. Preparing fire service professionals and their families for the implications of these large-scale natural disasters is necessary in advance.

The threat of **accidental disaster** depends significantly on the nature of your local economy and transportation system. For example, if your community has a significant chemical industry or chemicals are transported through it by truck or rail you are facing a possible accidental threat with catastrophic consequences. Helpful information is available through the Chemical Sector Information Sharing and Analysis Center (ISAC), Highway ISAC, and the Surface Transportation and

The threat of accidental disaster depends significantly on the nature of your local economy and transportation systems.

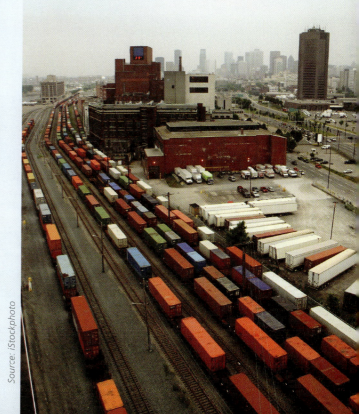

Source: iStockphoto

Public Transportation ISAC. See the CD for links to these organizations.

The ISAC Council provides information on several critical sectors and natural, accidental, or intentional threats to them. (See www.isaccouncil.org)

Local fire service agencies are probably the most familiar with the prominent sources of accidental threat in their community. In many cases, fire service agencies develop well-established relationships with private sector managers, often training and exercising with private sector security and safety personnel. Your fire service agency is a valuable collaborative partner in developing intelligence to meet the goal of preventing catastrophe.

Intentional threats are more difficult to monitor, and the role of fire service professionals in detecting intentional threats remains less defined. The sources of intentional threats are secretive. Further, without considerable care the attempt to collect intelligence regarding intentional threats can invade the civil liberties of innocent citizens. Martinez and McLoughlin are probably correct in asserting that more often than not, fire service professionals consume intelligence received from other homeland security agencies. ("The Fire Service and Counter-terrorism…") As they rightly add, there are many opportunities available to fire service professionals to develop information that others can investigate and analyze regarding intentional threats.

State and local first responder agencies consistently indicate they want increased effectiveness in intelligence sharing with the federal government. While this is a realistic concern, it is also true that local first responders often overestimate the capacity of the federal intelligence community to develop intelligence that is actionable at the local level.

In terms of the terrorist threat, clandestine and technological methods may identify when an attack has been authorized, the nature of the attack, and even the category of target. However, the precise method, date, and site of an attack is often the decision of a local cell. Unless the federal intelligence aligns with local intelligence, prevention is difficult.

A source of intelligence not always considered is the general citizenry.
Jonathan B. Tucker has written, "The vigilance of the Israeli public plays a key role in preventing terrorism. According to security experts, the average Israeli is highly aware of suspicious packages, individuals, and actions that could pose a threat to public safety and does not hesitate to notify the police. As a result, ordinary citizens foil more than 80%

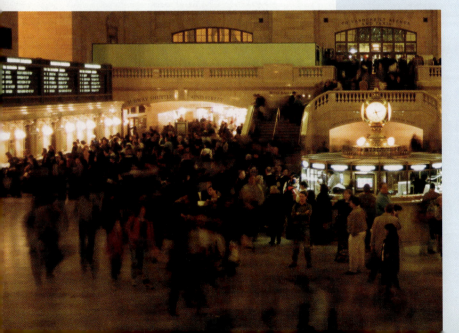

Grand Central Station, New York City
Source: Ablestock.com

of attempted terrorist attacks in Israel, including time bombs left by terrorists" (*Strategies for Countering Terrorism*).

Citizen complaints or leads have initiated several U.S. prosecutions for support of or conspiracy to terrorism. **Networking with the public, informing the public, and sharing information with the public is one of the most effective means for gathering information and proactively preventing catastrophe.** Moreover, as we noted in the Introduction, the public considers the fire service at the top of first responder agencies in terms of its members' approachability. Sometimes citizens provide vital information. Zacharias Moussaoui, who claims to have been involved in the 9/11 attacks, was arrested less than four weeks before the attack. A flight instructor became suspicious and reported him to the Immigration and Naturalization Service.

Good solid fire service work—with an eye on the broader context—is also a great source of intelligence. A case from Kings Park, New York, highlights the issues involved in passing along information to agencies in your collaborative network. The Kings Park Fire Department responded to an alarm in the spring of 2005 along the town's main street. The firefighters noticed items and documents during the operation that made them suspect a relationship to terrorist activity. They decided to pass on the information to their company officer who passed the same along to the Chief. The Chief spoke to the tenants and the fire investigators. The fire investigators also expressed concerns. The Chief and fire investigators then passed the same information along to the police, who notified detectives in the Intelligence Unit.

Ultimately, Immigration and Customs Enforcement (ICE) picked up the building occupants who were eventually deported. Yet, as Martinez and McLoughlin note, "It is not enough to pass on information with the hope that it will arrive at the best points of contact. Fire personnel must confirm that the matter is followed through. Not every item we note or see will lead to a major arrest; most information will be nonessential, but we are not in a position to make that call. If something does not appear correct or is perceived as a potential threat, report it" ("The Fire Service and Counterterrorism…"). Notice that Kings Park does not run a separate counterterrorism unit within its department. Nevertheless, the Chief and others involved followed up on the information sharing in a collaborative manner

Does your fire service agency have a protocol for managing citizen inputs to threat recognition?

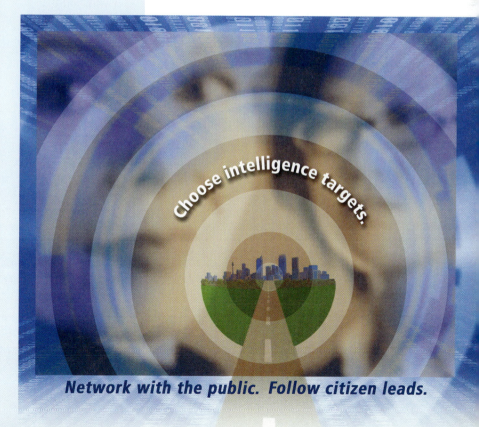

Choose intelligence targets.

Network with the public. Follow citizen leads.

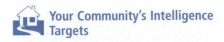

Your Community's Intelligence Targets

Does your fire service agency have an existing intelligence function? (circle one)

yes   no   I don't know

If no, it is not necessary to answer the following.

Does your fire service agency formally collaborate with the law enforcement intelligence function?

yes   no   I don't know

Have you ever received an intelligence briefing?

yes   no

Have you contributed data and information to an intelligence function?

yes   no

As a fire service professional, what do you perceive are the **top three priority targets** for your fire intelligence function:

___ Analysis of law enforcement intelligence for fire purposes
___ Arson investigation
___ Building inspections
___ Building Tactical Information database collection
___ Hazardous material identification and inventory
___ Hazardous material containment and mitigation
___ Organizing firewise communities
___ Support for Law Enforcement intelligence function
___ Other, please specify: _____
___ Other, please specify: _____

to make sure the information reached the correct authorities.

An additional example from Seattle demonstrates the importance of information sharing. An Engine Company with the Seattle Fire Department conducted an impromptu building inspection in April 2006. The inspection resulted from an observation of potential unsafe conditions at a building formerly used as a mosque. The inspection team found several hundred military chemical and biological hoods in the occupancy. Fire personnel recognized the circumstances as a potential indicator of terrorist activity and notified the FBI (Flynn, John).

Choosing your intelligence targets is—basically—deciding which risks are worth your regular attention.

Max Bazerman and Michael Watkins have tried to uncover why smart people and successful organizations so often fail to effectively manage predictable surprises. They have found a consistent pattern of **choosing the wrong priorities**. They explain,

"Prioritization failures arise when leaders and organizations recognize potential threats but do not deem them sufficient to warrant serious attention. The cognitive and organizational barriers to effective prioritizing are formidable. On the cognitive side, positive illusions and the tendency to discount the future, and thus underestimate the likelihood and impact of potential problems, loom as major barriers to effective prioritization. On the organizational side, the tendency to maintain the status quo, exacerbated by collective action problems or conflicts of interest, renders key people unwilling or unable to embrace the right set of priorities, with predictable results."

Deciding that catastrophic threats are appropriate intelligence targets should ensure regular attention, and regular attention will help combat the cognitive and organizational barriers that too often produce neglect.

Once your community's elected officials or senior public safety officials have recognized the need to think ahead about potential catastrophes, the intelligence function will need to translate wants and needs into specific requirements.

The CD includes a link to *Intelligence Essentials for Everyone* by Lisa Krizan. This document provides important guidance in developing a consumer-focused intelligence function. The CD also includes a Model Policy for criminal intelligence developed by the International Association of Chiefs of Police.

CHAPTER 3 — SHARE INFORMATION

COLLECTING DATA AND INFORMATION

Sources abound. Once you decide that catastrophic threats are an intelligence target, the operational issue is managing your sources of data and information.

With 24/7 cable news and the Internet the average citizen now has access to more information than most national intelligence agencies of twenty years ago. Access to information is not the problem. Picking and choosing is a serious problem.

Refining your target selection is fundamental to the collection process. Which catastrophes are either most likely or most consequential? **Apply a risk formula** to make a choice that is right for your community. Which catastrophes are most important for you to monitor? Which catastrophic risks are already being monitored elsewhere by others?

Your local law enforcement agency, public health agency, emergency management agency, or private sector organizations may already monitor many natural and accidental risks. If so, it is probably more efficient to **establish collaborative relationships** with these agencies to collect intelligence on those risks.

Many non-fire service organizations also monitor intentional risks. Think tanks, university research centers, insurance companies, and private security organizations are all involved in tracking computer hacking, hate crimes, terrorism, and other intentional threats. Working with these organizations may help extend whatever resources your fire service agency can apply.

For example, if you have chosen to focus on terrorist capabilities following are a few open sources that may be very helpful.

What capabilities have terrorist organizations demonstrated? The National Counter Terrorism Center provides an online Worldwide Incidents Tracking System (http://wits.nctc.gov/). This system allows you to research patterns that might have particular implications for your local community. A report providing an overview of global patterns is also available. A similar database is provided by the Institute for Counter Terrorism (www.ict.org.il). 💿 Links to these are available on the CD.

💿 Also available on your CD is the US

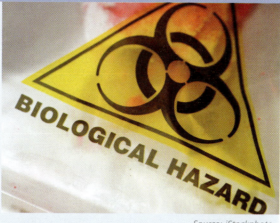

Source: iStockphoto

What sources of information do you find most helpful for your current assignments?

_____
_____
_____
_____
_____
_____

Do any of these include information on potential catastrophic threats?

_____
_____
_____
_____
_____
_____

Likelihood x *Consequences* = *Risk*

$$Likelihood = Threat \begin{cases} \times\ Vulnerability\ if\ \underline{\quad} \\ \text{\small(state conditions)} \\ /\ Vulnerability\ if\ \underline{\quad} \\ \text{\small(state conditions)} \end{cases}$$

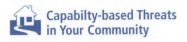

Capabilty-based Threats in Your Community

Please complete the following sentences:

Based on my current understanding of terrorist methods I perceive the most commonly used capability is:

_____

_____

I have

___ high confidence

___ some confidence

___ no confidence

in my answer.

Based on my current understanding of terrorist intentions I perceive the most dangerous terrorist capability for my community is:

_____

_____

I have

___ significant confidence

___ some confidence

___ no confidence

in my answer.

Based on my current understanding of intentional threats facing my community the most important question that I can work to answer with confidence is:

_____

_____

_____

Army's *A Military Guide to Terrorism in the 21st Century*. This document includes a chapter on current terrorist capabilities.

What new capabilities have terrorists demonstrated they wish to develop? According to the *Military Guide*, "Proliferation of weapons of mass destruction and the specter of their effects clearly amplify the dangers of a terrorist act. Information is readily available on many aspects of chemical, biological, radiological, nuclear, and conventional high yield explosives. Materiel for attempting the construction of WMD is easily accessible in the public domain. The knowledge and technological means of specialists to produce WMD is a shadowy area of science, crime, and intrigue available to the terrorist." Also on the CD is an article by Kate Marquis entitled, *Did 9/11 matter? Terrorism and Counterterrorism Trends: Present, Past, and Future*.

What do you need to know about these current or possible terrorist capabilities? Specifically, **how can your community take action to prevent or mitigate these capabilities?** The National Technical Information System provides a Homeland Security Information Center (http://www.ntis.gov/hs/) that provides detailed background on many terrorist capabilities. Other resources are available online from the Federation of American Scientists especially in regard to the use of Weapons of Mass Destruction (www.fas.org/terrorism/wmd)

Explicit questions are a good way to organize your approach to collecting data and information. What does your commanding officer want and need to know? How about the Chief? What questions do elected officials have? How about the general public? Identifying the right questions will narrow your search and make collection much more practical and productive.

Before proceeding, take a moment to complete the worksheet at left.

The Neighborhood Watch Model

To combat local terrorism the effective model is less James Bond and more Aunt Bea. Sheriff Taylor's and Opie's matriarch knew her neighbors, cared about them, and was both welcoming and curious about newcomers in the neighborhood. It is tough to be an effective terrorist in the midst of a caring community.

For over thirty years the National Sheriff's Association has sponsored local Neighborhood Watch programs. Today many of these local groups—sometimes in cooperation with the Department of Homeland Security's Citizen Corps program—have added the terrorist threat to their prevention goals. A **Neighborhood Watch** is a group of volunteers who are trained to be alert, recognize the symptoms and signals of various threats, and communicate effectively with each other and with law enforcement to prevent crime.

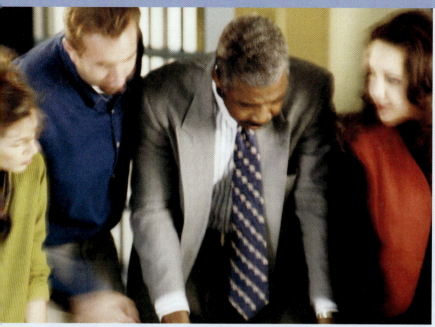
Source: PhotoDisc

As we noted in Chapter 1, **the public considers the fire service among the easiest of first responder professions to approach**, and many public safety programs in fire departments across the United States attest to this fact. Much of the fire service's public safety focus is on fire and accident prevention. Some observers in the profession suggest that community oriented policing provides a useful model for terrorism prevention in the fire service. Indeed, researchers interviewing and surveying fire service personnel in the Los Angeles and New York City fire departments contend that incorporating terrorism prevention into the fire service in a manner that engages the community means developing the ability of line staff, not just Chiefs and Captains, to elicit input from the community regarding suspicious situations (Welch; Flynn, John).

Strategic Intelligence Co-Laboratories

Many states and larger cities have established intelligence **fusion centers**. According to the August 2006 version of the U.S. Department of Justice and Department of Homeland Security *Fusion Center Guidelines*, one central question drives the guidelines for the organization and operation of fusion centers.

How can law enforcement, public safety, and private entities embrace a collaborative process to improve intelligence sharing and, ultimately, increase the ability to detect, prevent, and solve crimes while safeguarding our homeland?

Fusion centers are important formal mechanisms for sharing intelligence—both classified and open—for operational purposes.

Uncovering the intentional threat of terrorists almost always requires local know-how. Developing trusted networks and trusting relationships in the community is one of the best ways to collect the data and information that might expose an intentional threat. Of the following resources typical of many communities, **which ones do you think offer the most likely sources for useful information on terrorist threats?**

___ Religious Groups

___ Fraternal, Social, and Civic Groups

___ Real Estate Agents

___ Housing Managers

___ Storage Facility Managers

___ Transportation and Tourist Centers

___ Hotels

___ Businesses Selling Hazardous Materials

___ Industrial Facilities

___ Delivery Services

___ Print Shops

___ Inspectors and Code Enforcers

___ Facility License Records

___ Bar Employees

___ Colleges and Universities

___ Schools

___ Health Care Providers

___ Trash Collectors

___ Equipment Rental Companies

___ Taxi Services

CHAPTER 3 — SHARE INFORMATION

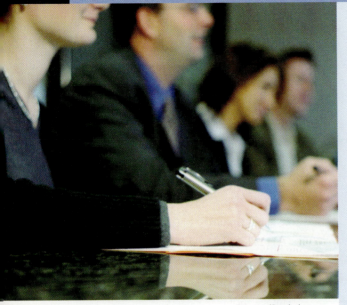

Source: iStockphoto

The fusion process encourages sharing of implicit knowledge, guesses, strategic leads, and good questions in a way formal communication systems can seldom achieve.

According to the Department of Homeland Security:

A **fusion center** is defined as a "collaborative effort of two or more agencies that provide resources, expertise, and information to the center with the goal of maximizing their ability to detect, prevent, investigate, and respond to criminal and terrorist activity." … Nontraditional collectors of intelligence, such as public safety entities and private sector organizations, possess important information (e.g., risk assessments and suspicious activity reports) that can be "fused" with law enforcement data to provide meaningful information and intelligence about threats and criminal activity. It is recommended that the fusion of public safety and private sector information with law enforcement data be virtual through networking and utilizing a search function. Examples of the types of information incorporated into these processes are threat assessments and information related to public safety, law enforcement, public health, social services, and public works.

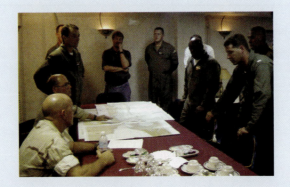

FEMA meeting
Source: DefenseLink

It is the fusion *process*—working together and meeting together—even more than the physical center itself that encourages the sharing of implicit knowledge, guesses, strategic leads, and good questions in a way that formal communications systems can seldom achieve. Fusion Centers become a collection mechanism simply by bringing people together who might otherwise not speak to one another. Fusion Centers often include representatives from area fire departments. The Arizona Fusion Center, called the Arizona Counter Terrorism Information Center (ACTIC), includes officers from eight fire departments in the state. Your CD contains a weblink providing more information. The focus of ACTIC is as an all-hazards, all crime, fusion center organization. The California State Terrorism Threat Assessment Center (STTAC) and Regional Terrorism Threat Assessment Centers (RTTAC) are all-hazards/all crime organizations. You may find it helpful to develop a similar local body focused on strategic intelligence.

Fusion Centers predominantly focus on counterterrorism, with only a few states including a multidisciplinary emphasis on all-hazards and all crimes. Counterterrorism is obviously important, but **the goal of preventing catastrophe requires data collection and information analysis of all catastrophic risks**. Managing your community's most serious risks with the resources

CHAPTER 3 — SHARE INFORMATION

available requires an authentically all-hazards approach to risk management.

A strategic intelligence co-laboratory offers an especially effective way to integrate intelligence gathering on natural, accidental, and intentional threats. In this way, a common strategic approach to all catastrophic risks is encouraged.

Some communities are hard-pressed to assign a sworn officer or any paid employee to strategic intelligence. A strategic intelligence co-laboratory is one way that auxiliary officers, or volunteers, or others organize to collect strategic intelligence under part-time supervision.

A weekly meeting of these volunteers—or even a monthly meeting with weekly teleconferences—is a practical way to begin developing a strategic intelligence function. A small investment made today is often much better than waiting to undertake a more ambitious plan later.

The International Association of Law Enforcement Intelligence Analysts is a good source of information and training. More information is available at www.ialeia.org.

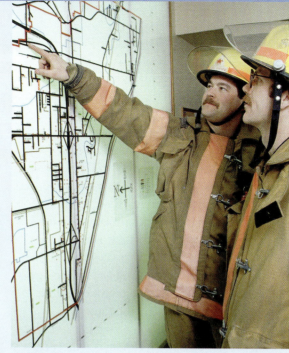

Source: Ablestock.com

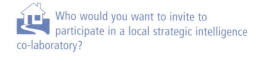

Who would you want to invite to participate in a local strategic intelligence co-laboratory?

A small investment made today is often better than waiting to undertake a more ambitious plan later.

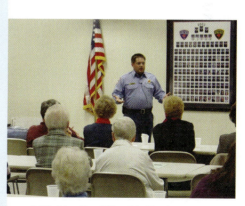

Public Education Officer Eric Vaughn meets with a seniors group.
Source: Bloomington Fire Department, Bloomington, IL

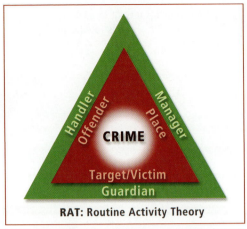

Source: The Home Office, Government of the United Kingdom

Offender: A person, organization, or other threat that endangers public safety

Target: A person or organization susceptible to harm from offenders

Place: A vulnerable location

ORGANIZE AND ANALYZE DATA AND INFORMATION

According to Russell Swenson of the Joint Military Intelligence College, "Successful intelligence analysis is a holistic process involving both 'art' and 'science.' Intuitive abilities, inherent aptitudes, rigorously applied skills, and acquired knowledge together enable analysts to work problems in a multi-dimensional manner, thereby avoiding the pitfalls of both scientism and adventurism. The former occurs when scientific methodology is excessively relied upon to reveal the 'truth;' the latter occurs when 'inspiration [is] unsupported by rigorous analysis.'" (*Bringing Intelligence About: Practitioners Reflect on Best Practices*)

Even if you choose only one intelligence target—for example intentional threats with catastrophic potential—and only assign a combination of volunteers and professionals equal to one full-time person, and even if you only access open sources, the flow of data and information will soon overwhelm you. **Before you can do anything with the information, you need to organize it.**

Collation

Organization means to take what is random and begin to make it relevant. This is usually accomplished by separating information into various **categories**. The categories are selected to reflect aspects of the problem that you are trying to solve.

If your problem is how to prevent catastrophe, and your focus is on intentional threats, you need to think through key elements of the problem and begin to use those key elements to categorize your information.

Every set of categories has its strengths and weaknesses. One of the reasons that intelligence agencies miss "connecting the dots" is because of how they define the problem. The problem definition results in organizing information so that an unanticipated threat does not easily emerge from the intelligence process. As a result, the dots themselves are not recognized.

Well-funded intelligence agencies try to avoid this "framing" limitation by organizing information using multiple models and different problem definitions. Many fire service agencies require only modest efforts, and remain conscious of the limitations of the problem-definition chosen.

One way to define the problem—and identify helpful organizational categories—is the **Routine Activity Theory** or **RAT**. This is a way of looking at problems first recognized in environmental criminology. The fire service provides an indirect crime prevention role through inspections that impede the rate of dilapidation in urban environments. **Think of an "offender" as any person or organization that endangers public safety** either through intentional action, as a terrorist, or through a failure to act, such as an organization storing, handling, or transporting hazardous materials in violation of fire codes or DHS regulations.

According to RAT three elements are necessary before a crime can happen:
1. **A target of interest to an offender is available.**
2. **The target is vulnerable, posing harm to public safety.**
3. **A likely and motivated offender is present.**

These three traditional categories of problem solving are very similar to the key elements of catastrophe prevention outlined above.

Some applications of RAT have expanded the three categories to six, as in the graphics shown on the facing page and at right.

But whether three or six, the RAT categories provide a framework that can be used to organize the information collected. What places have terrorists found interesting elsewhere? Does your community have such places? How accessible are those places? How can accessibility be better managed? Is there evidence of potential harmful intent? Actual harmful intent? Please use your CD to access more information on Routine Activity Theory. See *Opportunity Makes the Thief* by Felson and Clarke.

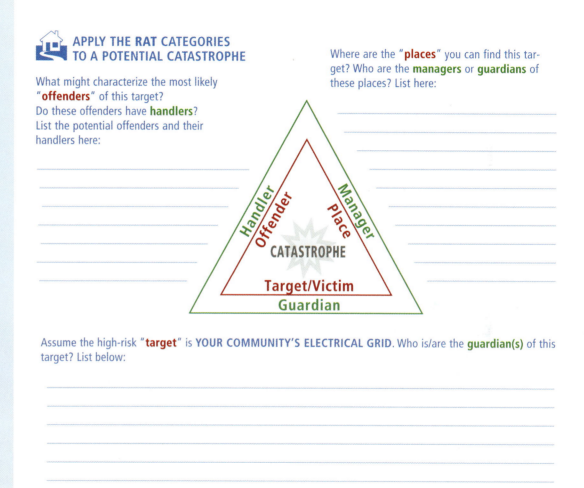

APPLY THE RAT CATEGORIES TO A POTENTIAL CATASTROPHE

What might characterize the most likely "**offenders**" of this target? Do these offenders have **handlers**? List the potential offenders and their handlers here:

Where are the "**places**" you can find this target? Who are the **managers** or **guardians** of these places? List here:

Assume the high-risk "**target**" is YOUR COMMUNITY'S ELECTRICAL GRID. Who is/are the **guardian(s)** of this target? List below:

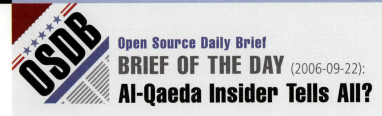

Open Source Daily Brief

BRIEF OF THE DAY (2006-09-22):
Al-Qaeda Insider Tells All?

A new book written by an individual claiming to be a former French spy inside Al-Qaeda is now available online and in many bookstores.

Written under the pseudonym Omar Nasiri, the book describes the intentions and capabilities of the Al Qaeda network during the late 1990s. According to Nasiri there was an ongoing effort to develop and deploy chemical, biological, and nuclear weapons. The book also describes the terrorist organization's training processes and tactical methods.

The *International Herald Tribune* asks, "But is it true?" The newspaper seems to conclude that the author's account may be mostly true.

Understanding an adversary's intentions and capabilities is obviously worth a great deal. The accuracy of such an understanding is difficult to determine in advance of an adversary taking action. One approach to evaluating the reliability of intelligence information is the 5x5 system. Recently the United Kingdom adapted this system for police intelligence gathering and analysis.

Under the 5x5 system a source of information — such as the Omar Nasiri memoir—can be assessed both in terms of the source providing the information and the nature of the information itself:

Source:

A. Always Reliable

B. Mostly Reliable

C. Sometimes Reliable

D. Unreliable

E. Source Untested

Information:

1. Known to be true without reservation

2. Known personally to the source but not to the person reporting

3. Not known personally to the source but corroborated

4. Cannot be judged

5. Suspected to be false.

Intelligence provided by an Always Reliable Source (A) consisting of information Known to be true (1) is tagged as A1 and is given much more attention than E5.

PREVENTION RELEVANCE: Prevention requires sharing information. The validity or reliability of information can be difficult to determine.

PREVENTION TECHNIQUES: Share Information: The 5x5 system was preceded by the so-called 4x4 system. There are many different thinking tools for assessing reliability. Find one that is well suited for your local condition.

PREVENTION THOUGHT: Share Information
What criteria do you informally use to assess validity? Can these informal criteria form the basis for a more explicit and formal system?

The Open Source Daily Brief is a service of the Institute for Preventive Strategies (©IPS). You can register to receive the OSDBs at www.preventivestrategies.net.

Validation

With the information organized, it is important to examine whether the information is valid. In some cases, this is mostly a matter of confirming facts and is often the case for natural or accidental threats. Yet, in the case of intentional threats, your ability to decide if something is right or wrong diminishes, meaning you need to assess for reliability. The known track record of the source, and the plausibility of the information, generally determine reliability. **Reliability is a standard that requires constant evaluation.** Information proven factually wrong is at the top of the list for removal from your collection unless exceptions apply.

You need to flag information included or excluded from your collection based on its reliability. Also, remove information from the collection informing your analysis that initially looked relevant to your problem, but is of uncertain reliability. In many cases, retaining such information outside the main collection is the right solution.

Similarly, periodically examine "reliable" information in the collection to determine if over time the source of information is, in fact, reliable.

A new source of information—especially seemingly implausible information—is often considered unreliable. What seems plausible can change over time. Traditional sources of information that helped in the past may "go cold" and become misleading. In either case, it is important that you self-consciously manage the influence of perceived reliability on your analysis.

When the same or similar information emerges from several different sources, this usually reinforces its reliability. If multiple sources independently report the same facts, or perceived facts, then you can usually

Validity and Reliability Testing

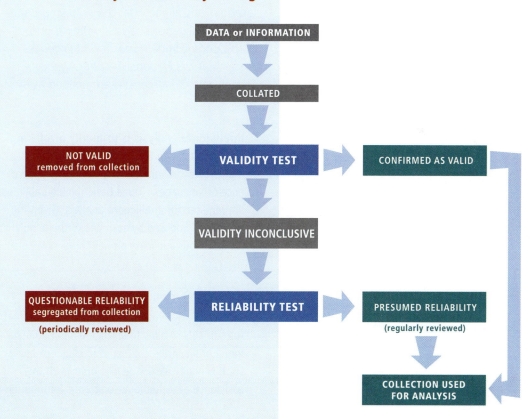

Give an example that cannot be assessed for validity:

_____
_____
_____
_____
_____
_____

🏠 Do you have a preference for or a particular expertise in one of the analytical skills described? If so, which one?

_____
_____
_____
_____
_____

Is one of the analytical skills especially difficult for you? If so, which one?

_____
_____
_____
_____
_____

Do you know someone who seems especially skilled at the form of analysis you find most difficult?

_____
_____
_____
_____
_____

assign greater reliability to the information. However, it is important to assess if your multiple sources are, in fact, independent. Or are they all repeating the same story of a single source? Separate origins for similar information is reassuring. Being sure of the separate origins is sometimes difficult.

Analytical Skills

With a collection of validated information organized to reflect your problem, you are ready to analyze the information. David T. Moore and Lisa Krizan of the Joint Military Intelligence College offer the following definition of intelligence analysis in their monograph *Core Competencies for Intelligence Analysis at the National Security Agency.* These same competencies are needed at the local level.

Intelligence analysis is primarily a thinking process; it depends upon cognitive functions that evolved in humans long before the appearance of language… Three basic thinking abilities are required for intelligence analysis. Given the limitations imposed by each one of them, only simultaneous application of all three may yield successful intelligence analysis.

Information Ordering:
This ability involves following previously defined rules or sets of rules to arrange data in a meaningful order. In the context of intelligence analysis, this ability allows people, often with the assistance of technology, to arrange information in ways that permit analysis, synthesis, and extraction of meaning. The arrangement of information according to certain learned rules leads the analyst to make conclusions and disseminate them as intelligence. A danger arises, however, in that such ordering is inherently limiting—the analyst may not look for alternative explanations because the known rules lead to a ready conclusion.

Pattern Recognition:
Humans detect patterns and impose patterns on apparently random entities and events in order to understand them, often doing this without being aware of it. Stellar constellations are examples of imposed patterns, while criminal behavior analysis is an example of pattern detection. Intelligence analysts impose or detect patterns to identify what targets are doing, and thereby to extrapolate what they will do in the future. Pattern recognition lets analysts separate "the important from the less important, even the trivial, and to conceptualize a degree of order out of apparent chaos." However, imposing or seeking patterns can introduce bias. Analysts may impose culturally defined patterns on random aggregates rather than recognize inherent patterns, thereby misinterpreting the phenomena in question.

Reasoning:
The ability to reason is what permits humans to process information and formulate explanations, to assign meaning to observed phenomena. It is by reasoning that analysts transform information into intelligence, in **these three ways**:

CHAPTER 3 — SHARE INFORMATION

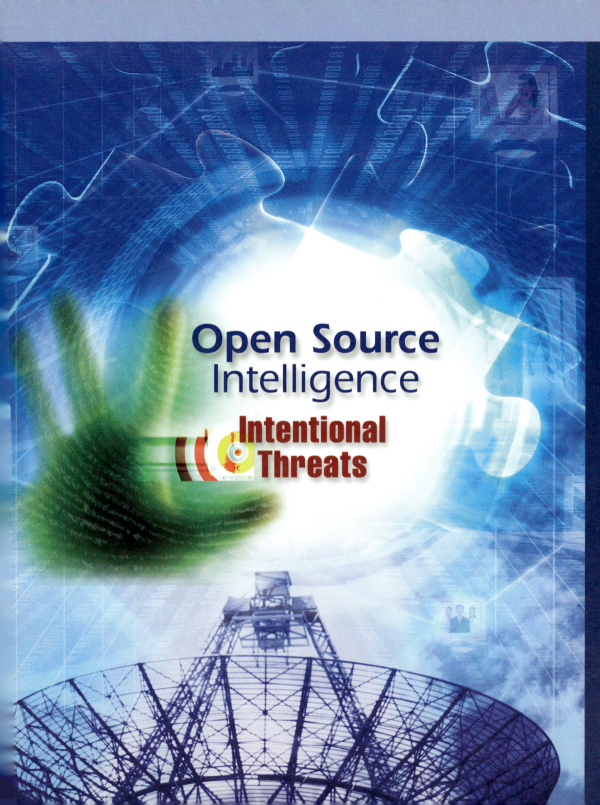

Open Source Intelligence
Intentional Threats

resources

Global
- Al-Jazeera, BBC, CNN-International
- State Department List of Foreign Terrorist Organizations
- National Counter Terrorism Center Worldwide Incidents Tracking System

Provides a sense of strategic context, terrorist methods, and potential trends.

National
- Major Media: Broadcast, Newspaper, and Periodical
- Southern Poverty Law Center-Intelligence Project
- Homeland Security conferences, courses, and books

Provides indicators of emerging threats and successful prevention strategies.

Regional
- Regional Media
- Economic development organizations
- State, County, and Local Transportation Agencies
- State, County, and Local public works, water works, and similar organizations
- Electric utilities
- Telecommunications Industry
- Farmers, agribusiness, and food sector
- Business associations, Labor Unions, and other existing cooperatives

Provides background on potential local targets and vulnerabilities.

Local
- News Media
- Neighborhood Associations
- Faith Based Organizations
- Citizen Complaints
- Community Policing

Provides data and information on potential threat capabilities.

Which form of analysis do you perceive is most commonly used in fire service work? Why?

___

Is the form of analysis you chose above also effective in preventing catastrophe? Why or why not?

___

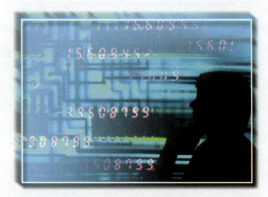

1. Induction:
Inductive reasoning combines separate fragments of information, or specific answers to problems, to form general rules or conclusions. For example, using induction, a child learns to associate the color red with heat and heat with pain, and then to generalize these associations to new situations. Rigorous induction depends upon demonstrating the validity of causal relationships between observed phenomena, not merely associating them with each other.

2. Deduction:
Deductive reasoning applies general rules to specific problems to arrive at conclusions. Analysts begin with a set of rules and use them as a basis for interpreting information. For example, an analyst who follows the nuclear weapons program of a country might notice that a characteristic series of events preceded the last nuclear weapons test. Upon seeing evidence that those same events are occurring again, the analyst might deduce that a second nuclear test is imminent. However, this conclusion would be made cautiously, since deduction works best in closed systems such as mathematics, making it of limited use in forecasting human behavior.

3. Abduction:
Abductive reasoning describes the thought process that accompanies "insight" or intuition. When the information does not match that expected, the analyst asks "why?," thereby generating novel hypotheses to explain given evidence that does not readily suggest a familiar explanation. For example, given two shipping manifests, one showing oranges and lemons being shipped from Venezuela to Florida, and the other showing carnations being shipped from Delaware to Colombia, abductive reasoning is what enables the analyst to take an analytic leap and ask, "Why is citrus fruit being sent to the worldwide capital of citrus farming, while carnations are being sent to the world's primary exporter of that product? What is really going on here?" Thus, abduction relies on the analyst's preparation and experience to suggest possible explanations that must then be tested. Abduction generates new research questions rather than solutions.

Self-awareness of Hypotheses

Fundamental to disciplined thinking is taking responsibility for your hypotheses. Producing a tentative explanation that you want to test is creating a hypothesis. In fire investigation this is an ongoing process of problem solving. Investigators generate hypotheses which they then test-out, seeking evidence to support or deny their tentative explanation.

In sorting through and analyzing information for intelligence purposes, it is especially important to be self-aware of your hypotheses. Write down your tentative explanation. If possible write it down in the form of a question that can be denied. Work as hard to deny it as to confirm it.

Explicit—and deniable—hypotheses are the best way to ensure that your insights are tested with scientific rigor. This is most likely to achieve the right balance of art and science in intelligence analysis.

PRODUCE INTELLIGENCE PRODUCTS

The purpose of the intelligence process is to help consumers of intelligence better understand their situation and make decisions. When the situation includes the potential for catastrophe, focus the intelligence process on providing strategic intelligence to enable these consumers to make decisions that prevent or mitigate natural, accidental, or intentional catastrophe.

For the purpose of preventing or mitigating catastrophe who are your consumers of intelligence?

Before proceeding, take a moment to complete the worksheet on the right side of this page.

The purpose of intelligence is to support effective decision-making. **The consumer of intelligence is someone who needs to make a decision.** Some decisions—especially in the private sector—may be closely held.

Other key decisions may be made through the democratic process. The needs of your consumer should influence how you develop and package the intelligence product.

Intelligence products are traditionally delivered to a very small number of consumers. This is, in part, necessary to protect confidential sources and methods utilized in collecting the intelligence.

The need for confidentiality is reduced if your intelligence product primarily uses open sources that focus largely on strategic, rather than tactical or evidentiary, purposes. If your sources and methods are transparent and open, there is less cause to restrict access to your intelligence product.

Nevertheless, **each consumer has different needs**. Each consumer plays different roles in the decision-making process. If your intelligence product is to help, it must reflect the sense of priority and the real needs of each consumer. What the mayor needs is often different from what the Fire Chief needs and what the engineer needs is different from what the fire inspector needs. What will each consumer recognize as relevant to his or her role?

Just as you must make choices in narrowing your collection of information and data, you must also recognize your priority consumers of intelligence.

For the purpose of preventing or mitigating catastrophe who are your consumers of intelligence? Who is likely to be involved in making decisions that could influence the ability of your community to prevent or mitigate catastrophe?

___ Senior Fire Service Officials
___ Fire Service Rank-and-File
___ Senior Local Police Officials
___ Local Police Rank-and-File
___ State Law Enforcement Officials
___ Federal Law Enforcement Officials
___ Senior Public Health Officials
___ Public Health Rank-and-File
___ Senior Public Works Officials
___ Public Works Rank-and-File
___ Senior Emergency Management Officials
___ Emergency Management Rank-and-File
___ Other Intelligence Officials
___ Local Elected Officials
___ State Elected Officials
___ Federal Elected Officials
___ Senior Hospital Management
___ Owners of Private Sector Critical Infrastructure (power utilities, telecommunications, transportation systems, etc.)
___ News Media
___ Neighborhood Leaders
___ Faith Community Leaders
___ General Public
___ Other, please specify: _____

___ Other, please specify: _____

Packaging the Product

Do you know **your consumer's preferences**? Do they want one-pagers or research papers? Do they prefer text or pictures? Do they want a discussion or a presentation? How do they consume? When do they consume?

_____
_____
_____
_____
_____
_____
_____

Does your consumer want you to draw implications and suggest conclusions, or do they see your role as presenting organized information that they are to analyze?

_____
_____
_____
_____

Do they see you as a partner in decision-making or just a vendor of processed information?

_____
_____
_____

Does your consumer respond best to a constant flow of information or periodic summaries?

_____
_____
_____
_____

Are you packaging the intelligence product just for your consumer or are you crafting a product that your consumer will feed to other consumers?

_____
_____

How does your consumer make decisions? How can you deliver an intelligence product that will best support that decision-making process?

_____
_____
_____
_____

What is your consumer's preexisting orientation to the issue?

_____
_____
_____

Do they already give priority to preventing catastrophe?

_____
_____

Do they tend to give greater attention to one threat over another?

_____
_____

Do they discount future threats in order to focus on immediate threats?

_____
_____

If you serve in an intelligence role, you almost certainly have an immediate consumer. What does he or she need? Why is this person your immediate consumer? Does your consumer in turn supply intelligence to another consumer? How are the needs of the ultimate consumer different from your immediate consumer?

Credibility and Effectiveness

Whatever the package, the content of an intelligence product—especially its accuracy and utility over time—determines whether there is any real consumption of your product.

There is always ongoing tension between giving your consumer what he or she wants, and what you perceive is accurate. This is a classic problem of intelligence production and consumption. Sherman Kent, a long-time CIA analyst and one of the founding theorists of intelligence addressed this issue. In the following, **"Warners"** are the producers of intelligence, **"Warnees"** are the consumers.

> Warners know Warnees are hard to convince. They will not be warned by a hint. The thing that will really jolt them into being warned is for the Warner to push his conclusions beyond what his evidence will legitimately support. This is seldom done for good reason. It ain't honest. It ain't prudent.
>
> Warnees know all about the Warners' tendency to overwarn. And also about their fallibility.

The Warners' credibility declines with warnings that turn out to be false alarms. And in the event that the Warners once hurt by a false alarm fail to warn of an important event, their credibility may be cooked for good.

In face of uncertainty and aware of the CYA attitude of the Warners, Warnees make their own judgment of [the criteria for] warnability.

Such then is the unhappy psychological relationship between those who guard the health—even the life of the state.

This is reality. **The producer of intelligence must do his or her best to serve the needs of the consumer, but at the same time must be disciplined in avoiding over-statement or understatement.**

Producers of intelligence are a bit like a struggling but idealistic organic farmer. You desperately want the consumer to buy, but you are only going to sell what you think is good for the consumer.

Kent went ahead to offer **three suggestions for a healthy relationship between producers and consumers of intelligence:**

- Care on the part of Warners not to overload the circuits.
- Care on the part of Warnees not to develop too much callousness.
- Above all, more talk between the two.

CONSUME INTELLIGENCE PRODUCTS

Many fire service officers will contribute to intelligence products. Few will produce intelligence products. Most should be consumers of intelligence products. **What are the characteristics of an effective consumer?**

- **Communicate what you need and why you need it.** Identify and specify your intelligence targets. Take responsibility for focusing the intelligence process to best serve you. Be conscious of the trade-offs in choosing some priorities and excluding others.

- **Communicate how you want intelligence packaged and why.** Describe the needs of down-stream consumers.

- **Be self-aware of your existing biases and communicate these** to the producers of intelligence. Attempt to step outside those biases in your consumption. Try something new.

- **Ask questions.** Especially seek clarification regarding the reliability of the data and information that have informed the analysis.

- **Offer feedback.** Tell the producers what is especially helpful to your decision-making and why.

- **Take into consideration the needs of other consumers and the resources applied** to gathering, analyzing, and producing intelligence. Recognize the limitations of the producers of intelligence.

- **Make time to regularly consume intelligence in a thoughtful way.** Intelligence —especially strategic intelligence—is not usually a fast food. It is much more like an intense conversational dinner. You probably will not do it every day. But make time for it on a specific calendar.

The more consumer-friendly your product the more likely it will have influence on actual decisions.

SHARE INFORMATION:
Chapter Review

What is the difference between strategic intelligence and tactical intelligence?

The intelligence process is described differently depending on purpose and organization, even though the functions are usually similar. What are the five steps in the intelligence process summarized as C-COP-C?

What is a capability-based threat analysis? How does this differ from more traditional threat analysis?

What is an Open Source?

What is the principal difference between a capability-based threat assessment using open sources and the typical contents of a criminal intelligence file?

Why are sources of catastrophic threat an appropriate intelligence target?

What is an important technique to focus and limit the range of collecting data and information? Why is it important to focus and limit collecting?

How can the Routine Activity Theory be utilized to organize data and information? What is the danger of using this organizational framework?

Moore and Krizan identify three basic thinking abilities that are part of intelligence analysis. What are they?

What are key considerations in developing an effective intelligence product?

What are the principal characteristics of an effective intelligence consumer?

CHAPTER 3 — SHARE INFORMATION   83

APPLY WHAT YOU HAVE LEARNED

Use your CD to access the Information Sharing Advanced Exercise. Select the **Chapter 3** Certificate Course link located in the Online Exercises section of your CD.

It is now 12 months before a planned terrorist attack. As a Senior Captain in the San Luis Rey® Fire Department you are assigned the task of developing a strategic information plan that can be used to protect, deter, or preempt an imminent threat.

Utilizing the principles of Sharing Information presented in this workbook can you determine your informational needs, collect and evaluate the right information, and share it with your collaboration network? There is too much information available, **choices will be required**. The terrorists have been actively planning and collecting information.

Note: If you have already enrolled in the Homeland Security Terrorism Prevention Certificate Course for Fire Service Professionals (©IPS) you can go directly to the exercise by using the Online Exercises Direct Access links on your CD or by typing this URL into your browser's address window:

www.preventivestrategies.net/go/ mhfs-adv-ex-share-info

For first time access, use this initial URL:
www.preventivestrategies.net/go/ mhfs-enroll

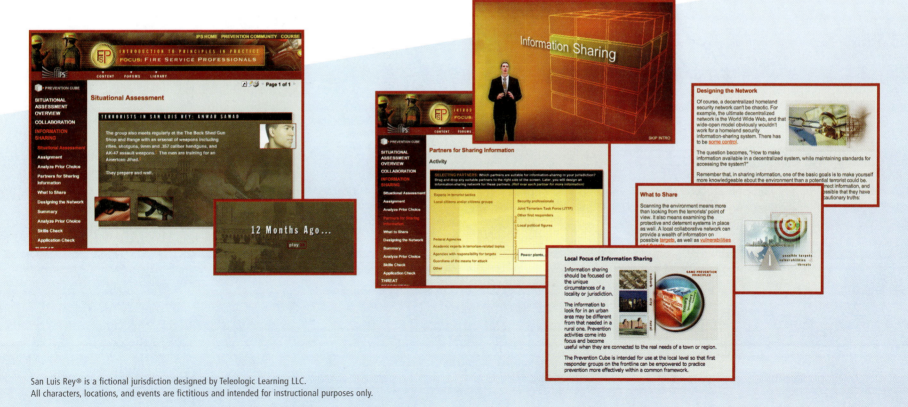

San Luis Rey® is a fictional jurisdiction designed by Teleologic Learning LLC.
All characters, locations, and events are fictitious and intended for instructional purposes only.

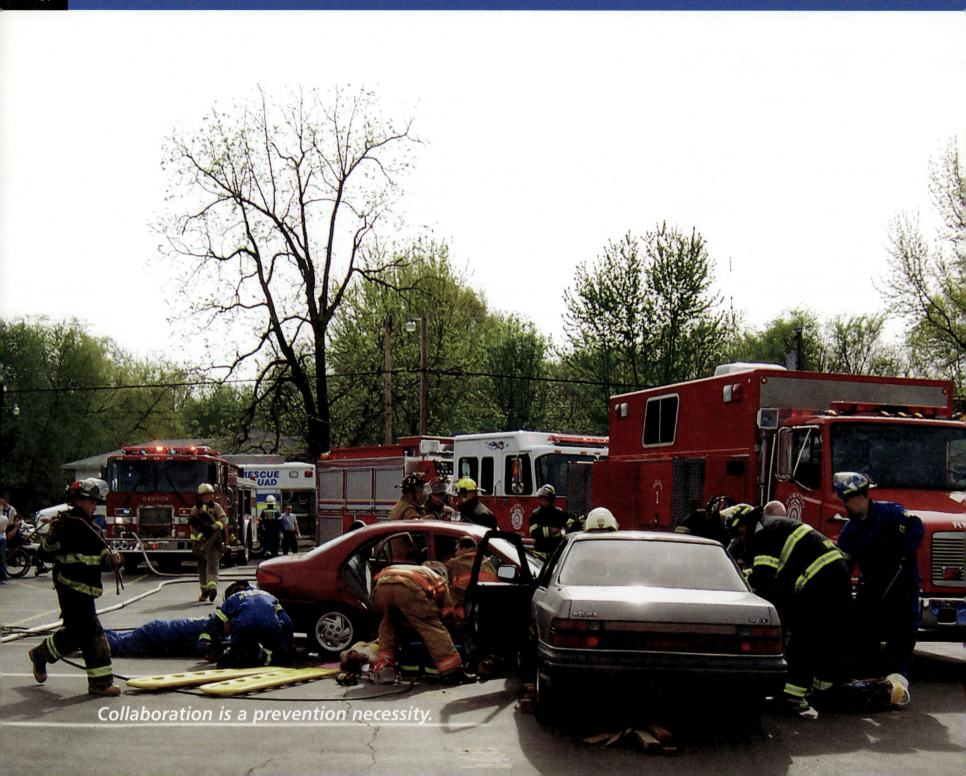
Collaboration is a prevention necessity.

Collaborate

✓ **In this chapter you will learn:**
- How to define collaboration.
- How to design collaboration to advance your goals.
- How the collaboration process works.
- How to conduct a self-evaluation using the Coleman Collaboration Equation.
- How to evaluate potential collaborators using the Coleman Collaboration Equation.
- How to apply collaboration to information sharing.
- How to apply collaboration to target identification.
- How to think about regional collaboration.
- How to engage collaborative agreements.

The story of Noah and the great flood is one of the oldest examples of preparing for catastrophe. According to Genesis, the ability to anticipate the disastrous event was due to divine "intelligence." The same intelligence source provided very specific instructions to manage the risk. Noah and his family had a limited time to complete a huge construction and animal gathering project.

Our intelligence sources are unlikely to be as unerring. But like Noah, we will need many others to help us respond effectively to the risks we face.

We cannot expect to receive divine forewarnings about catastrophes, whether natural, accidental, or intentional. Our efforts require humans working together to develop insights into community vulnerabilities, while planning for the elimination or mitigation of those vulnerabilities. **Collaboration involves sharing information and collectively analyzing it to extract intelligence about risks to the community.**

Most local first responder agencies do not have a separate intelligence unit. But fire service agencies share an interest in developing strategic intelligence on vulnerabilities in their community. Sharing strategic intelligence increases your ability to respond effectively to emergency incidents by understanding key information about the location. Vulnerabilities in any community cut across public and private lines as well as different public disciplines.

Your fire service agency almost certainly cannot collect and analyze all the strategic intelligence necessary to prepare for catastrophes. Collaboration is a key component of any attempt to prepare for catastrophic events.

Emergency management agencies have information and experience regarding all types of threats. Public health agencies are usually the experts on pandemic and similar health

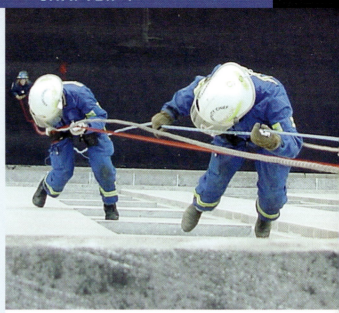

You can't do it alone.

FACING PAGE: *Sangamon County Rescue Squad, New Berlin Fire Department, and other Central Illinois agencies collaborate on training and emergency response.*

Above: *Sangamon County Rescue Squad engaged in high angle rescue training, Springfield, IL*

Source: Photos by Jerry McKay

> How do you currently use your network to solve professional problems?

threats. The private sector owns most of the infrastructure on which the health and wealth of your community depends. State, county, or local public works agencies manage most of the rest. Law enforcement agencies have expertise in preempting intentional threats.

White House policy, Congressional legislation, Department of Homeland Security regulations, and many DHS grant requirements all call for multi-agency, inter-governmental, private-public, and regional collaboration. Effective collaboration is fundamental to effective threat recognition, information sharing, and efforts to prevent or mitigate catastrophe.

DEFINING COLLABORATION

"Collaboration" has many different meanings. Sometimes people talk about collaboration when they just mean imposing a traditional command-and-control structure on non-traditional partners.

Real collaboration is **a self-interested recognition that cooperation between independent organizations is mutually helpful**. Given American traditions of separated and limited power, real collaboration may be the only practical way to achieve a coordinated approach to preventing catastrophe.

The Founding Fathers wrote the Constitution of the United States to limit centralized power. The American tradition of separation of powers—and competing power centers—is deeply woven into local, county, and state governments. The private sector is suspicious of government intrusion. One of the reasons all of this works so well is that U.S. political institutions reflect what seems to be a side of human nature that is very protective of turf. Because freedom is important to us, we resist outside interference.

However, many outsiders note that Americans are nearly unique in enthusiasm for voluntary organizations. We cooperate on ambitious public endeavors with minimum government involvement. Even as we resist outside pressure to conform, we are expert in self-generating cooperative ventures. We are a collaborative culture. We are predisposed to this essential element of preventing catastrophe.

Collaboration is the art of establishing a network of strategic partnerships or alliances in order to achieve a mutually desirable goal, in this particular case, preventing catastrophe.

Look at each of the key terms:

Art of establishing a network of strategic partnerships or alliances: Setting up partnerships requires work and finesse. While many preparedness officials accept catastrophe prevention as their responsibility, the private sector does not necessarily believe they play such a role. Whether recognized or not, everyone plays a role in prevention. Practitioners need to enlist both public and private partners to collaborate in this effort.

Network: A network is a group of partners working together. A network is different from many other forms of partnership. In a well-functioning network, the relationships are non-hierarchical, non-linear, and multi-layered. A network is multi-nodal. This means there are many places where sub-networks in the overall network overlap. Because of the multi-nodal nature of a network, a traditional command-and-control system is not necessary and can even undermine the efficiency of the network. Human networks are usually most effective when there is a strong sense of shared purpose and mutually understood goals across the network.

Strategic Partnership: Strategic partners focus on long-term goals and mutual advantage through an enduring network of collaborators (partners). A strategic partnership is usually built upon shared trust and respect, which allows effective movement toward common goals and purposes. Even where trust and respect are in doubt, a strategic partnership reflects mutual needs and mutual benefits.

Mutually Desirable Goal: Everyone has an interest in preventing catastrophe. But not everyone may feel they have a role in the work. **The goal must be highlighted** so everyone accepts that they should work toward it through lasting partnerships.

In "The Cycle of Preparedness: Establishing a Framework to Prepare for Terrorist Threats" William Pelfrey defines collaboration as, **"Agencies, organizations, and individuals from many tiers of public and private sectors, working, training, and exercising together for the *common purpose* of preventing terrorist threats to people or property."**

Collaboration extends across public organizations to private sector entities. In a true collaboration there is a **shared sense of**

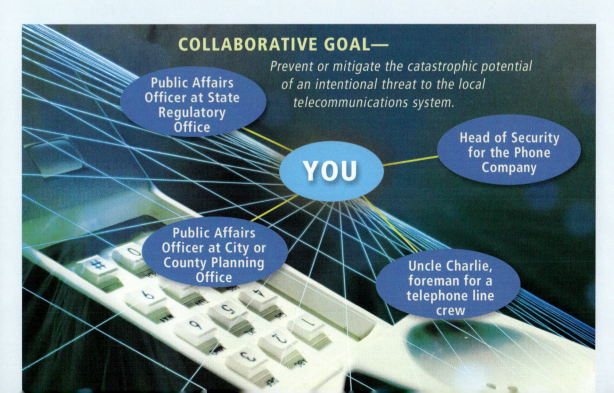

COLLABORATIVE GOAL—
Prevent or mitigate the catastrophic potential of an intentional threat to the local telecommunications system.

- Public Affairs Officer at State Regulatory Office
- Head of Security for the Phone Company
- YOU
- Public Affairs Officer at City or County Planning Office
- Uncle Charlie, foreman for a telephone line crew

At left is an example of a first-layer collaborative network. Each of these network partners may help you identify other network partners.

Where would you go first?

_____
_____
_____
_____
_____

CHAPTER 4 — COLLABORATE

You are already part of a network. To collaborate means to be self-conscious in using your network to achieve a goal.

Use the diagram at left and the space below to **map out your goal-oriented network.** Focus on preventing what you consider the highest priority catastrophic threat facing your community. **Try to go at least two layers deep.** *(Customize the diagram as needed.)*

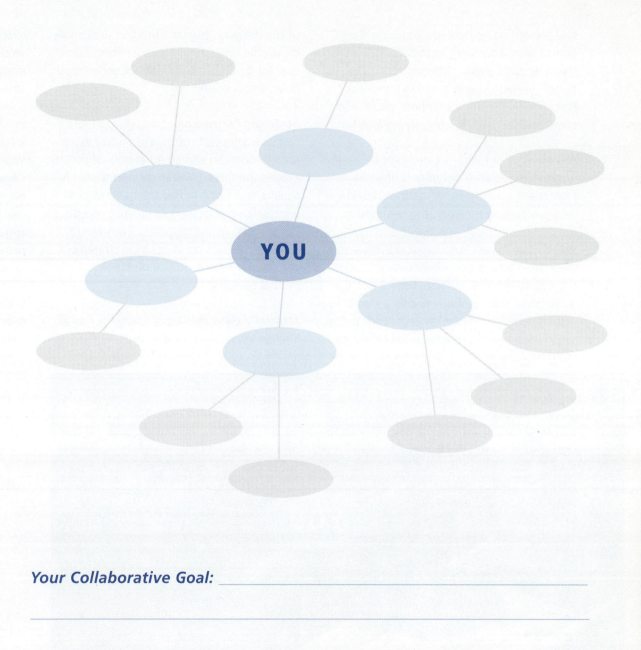

Your Collaborative Goal: _____

responsibility, uniform preparation, and a broad strategic partnership.

Importance of Collaboration

Collaboration is the foundation of effective prevention. Good collaboration establishes far-reaching networks and reduces the stove-piping effect. Information flows more efficiently through networks and is more likely to reach those who can act on it.

One way to recognize the importance of collaboration is to observe our adversaries. Al Qaeda calls on other Islamic fundamentalist groups to carry out attacks in a common purpose. They get intelligence information from a network of local sympathizers and informal partners. Al Qaeda makes deals with potential partners in many countries to provide safe houses in which to hide while they plan attacks. Collaboration is a central part of our adversary's ability to survive and operate.

RAND analysts John Arquilla, Dave Ronfeldt, and Michele Zanini point out, **"It takes a network to fight a network."** Without collaboration across government agencies, organizations, and the private sector, our adversaries hold a significant advantage.

Please access your CD to read Arquilla, Ronfeldt, and Zanini's article, "Networks, Netwars, and Information Age Terrorism."

Advantages of Collaboration

Collaboration enhances your ability to prevent and mitigate natural, accidental, and intentional threats. Forming purposeful alliances with the broader community accomplishes several objectives, including:

Improved information flow: Information flows easier through a network. When one channel is blocked, other channels will open to let it flow. For example, consider US efforts to cut off Al Qaeda's ability to communicate. Since October 2001, Osama bin Laden's group can no longer freely talk via cell phone for fear that our intelligence agencies are listening. Likewise, satellite phones are no longer used. Al Qaeda has resorted to handwritten notes via carriers, the Internet, and even certain media outlets. Despite our best efforts to stop the information flow, Al Qaeda continually finds alternative methods. Similarly, information can and should move through a variety of channels rather than just through a central hub, such as a CIA or FBI information clearinghouse.

Access to previously untapped sources in the private and public sectors: Collaboration can lead to many potential partners and, consequently, better information. Potential partners come from many places. The FBI's InfraGard® program is a good example. Recognizing that the federal government could not protect the Internet infrastructure alone, they assembled a group of partners to help prevent cybercrime. The collaborative network now has more than 19,000 members.

Broad acceptance and participation from others: Collaborating allows the community to participate and contribute to the effort, which helps unify and move more people towards the goal of preventing catastrophe. Clarence Harmon believes communities are more than willing to participate on a broad scale, "If the citizens are involved in the process of defending the nation and themselves, they will be empowered to prepare for and manage an array of scenarios." (*Turning a Popular War into a Populist War: Preparing the American Public for Terrorism*)

Flexibility to adjust to individual situations: A collaborative network provides flexibility. Partners who offer the most useful skills or information are consulted based on timing and specific needs. For example, in the online Introductory Exercise, it is important to speak with the Sheriff's Department about the motor carrier safety check, but it is also important to know that DAL Chemical can track the missing truck with a GPS system. In a non-collaborative situation, no one would consider calling DAL Chemical.

These advantages apply whether the threat is natural, accidental, or intentional; and whether the threat is catastrophic or not.

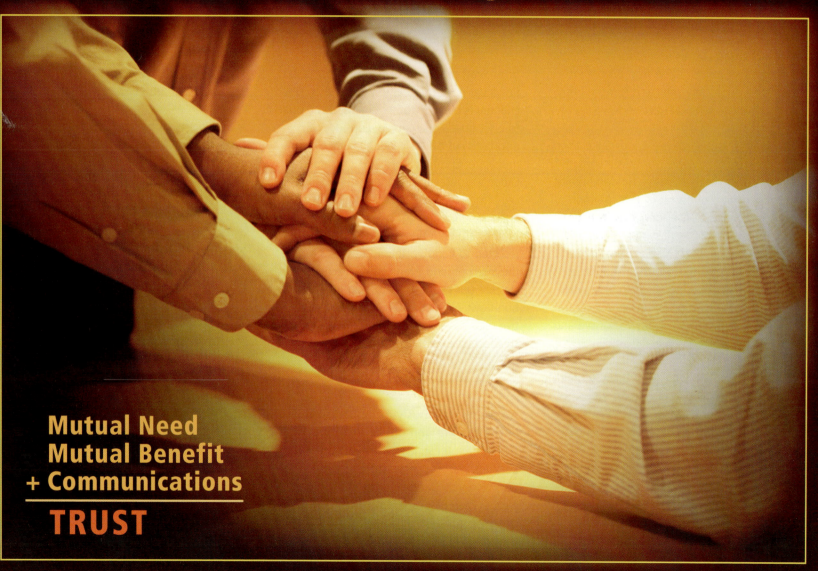

Collaboration and Change

Without collaboration, prevention is little more than a matter of luck. Before investing in collaboration, however, it is important to recognize the challenges involved. For example, in most communities, preparedness professions are not accustomed to collaborating among themselves, let alone with the broader community. It is uncommon for firefighters and law enforcement to meet regularly at the department or individual level to discuss issues that might benefit both. In some communities, police and fire may even see each other as competitors for the same resources.

Collaboration is not easy. It may not seem natural. In the beginning, it can even seem like a waste of time. However, over the long-term it is usually a necessary step in a realistic effort to prevent catastrophe.

COLLABORATION PROCESS

In *Governing by Network* Stephen Goldsmith and William Eggers argue that the future of government requires networking. The most important advantage of government-by-networking is allowing the agency to focus on what it does best while letting others add to the service or product to make it even better. Creating a network of collaborative partners can produce a similar effect in preventing catastrophe.

Building a network of collaborative partners is a significant task requiring a good deal of effort. However, the effort is well worth it if it prevents catastrophe. To begin creating a network of collaborators it is helpful to break the process into parts:

- Choosing collaborative goals.

- Designing a collaborative network to meet those goals.

- Selecting strategic partners within the network who can help achieve the goals.

Collaborative Goals

The National Strategy for Homeland Security identifies six major initiatives for domestic counterterrorism. First among them reads, "Improve intergovernmental law enforcement coordination."

The entire *National Strategy* is available on your CD.

Further, the strategy states: "To meet the terrorist threat, **we must increase collaboration and coordination**—in law enforcement and prevention, emergency response and recovery, policy development and implementation—so that public and private resources are better aligned to secure the homeland." **These federal goals provide a starting point for local level collaborative goals.** Fire service professionals must customize

---

Do you have an example of previously using collaboration to solve a fire service problem? If so, please describe it.

Why do individuals and organizations discount opportunities to collaborate?

🏠 What do you believe should be the goals for collaboration in your community in order to prevent or mitigate catastrophe?

_____
_____
_____
_____
_____
_____
_____
_____
_____
_____
_____
_____
_____

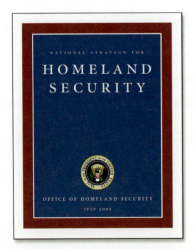

them to meet the specific needs of the local or state jurisdiction before implementation.

How can you tailor the goals to meet the needs of a specific jurisdiction or agency? Goldsmith and Eggers suggest some **key principles for determining goals:**

Determine the important public value. What public good is served? Answering this question helps establish policy goals and determine with whom to collaborate.

Do not define the problem or answer based on historical processes alone. The way of doing business in the past should not determine how and with whom to collaborate. Nor should current or past organizational structure dictate how to collaborate. Instead, the new possibilities that emerge from a collaborative network should guide thinking in how to resolve a problem.

Make the collaborative network design fit your desired outcome. The new network must complement and work towards the organization's goals.

With these principles in mind, your network of partners should be able to build off the federal goals for collaborating to prevent catastrophe at the local level.

What do you believe should be the goals for collaboration in your community in order to prevent or mitigate catastrophe?

DESIGNING A COLLABORATIVE NETWORK

Once you define the goals, begin the process of building the collaborative network:

- **Design the network.**

- **Select strategic partners for the network.**

- **Maintain the network.**

Designing the Network

Designing a collaborative network around the community's needs or goals requires a commitment to building social capital among the members of the community involved in protecting vulnerable locations or activities. Your goal is to prevent or mitigate catastrophe. You have identified those aspects of your community most vulnerable to different kinds of catastrophic threats. These key vulnerabilities—the water system, electrical system, food chain, health system, or whatever—begin to suggest potential collaborative partners.

What kind of information do you need? What kind of analysis do you need? What kind of operational cooperation do you need? What kind of joint training and planning do you need? Answering these questions will begin to define the strategic partners you need.

People are a crucial consideration. The collaboration effort may never get off the ground without certain people involved. Perhaps a few well-connected individuals, or groups, are available who can quickly activate the network by bringing a variety of private and/or public sector influentials into the collaboration effort. These key people might also lend the kind of credibility that encourages broad participation.

The type of collaborative network requires some thought. Goldsmith and Eggers offer some questions to ask when deciding what type to choose:

What do you want the network to do?

Will it deliver a service or provide information or something else?

With regard to preventing terrorism, it could be any combination of things depending on local needs.

Is the need ongoing or one-time?
For prevention, the network will need to be ongoing. However, there may be instances where it can be a temporary solution as well.

What is the relative importance of accountability versus flexibility?

The goal is to strike a balance between the government's responsibility for preventing an attack and letting collaborative partners perform functions for which they are better suited. The trick here is to use collaborative partners to enhance the government's ability to prevent terrorism while not shifting ultimate responsibility to anyone other than the appropriate agency.

Selecting Strategic Partners

Once your collaborative network defines its goals, **the next step is to select partners who bring strategic value into the mix**. Before bringing in partners, however, a self-check is necessary. A review of internal relationships is helpful to ensure the agency's readiness and capability for developing long-term partnerships.

Answering the following questions helps when selecting strategic partners:

- Who will effectively help achieve the long-term goals?
- What types of organizations or individuals can help?
- Are they in the private or public sector?
- Should non-profit or community-based groups be involved?
- What functions need performing?

In its basic form, the Incident Command System (ICS) provides a modular and scalable structure that supports five essential management functions in emergency response: command, planning, operations, logistics, and finance/administration (Bigley and Roberts). Moreover, the design of ICS, with its allowance for Unified Command, Area Command, and Unified Area Command, recognizes the importance of managing a network of response agencies and adapting the response effort as an emergency develops. For instance, the U.S. Fire Administration's Incident Management Team (IMT) program uses the ICS to provide command and control infrastructure with established teams of specialists during emergencies starting at the smallest, local unit and escalating according to the scale of the emergency to the state and national levels. See the CD for an IMT link.

The Exotic Newcastle Disease (END) outbreak in California in 2002–2003 provides a good example of the value of ICS to emergency response, and speaks directly to the importance of a strategic approach to collaboration. END is a highly contagious and generally fatal disease to poultry. The California outbreak was contained through collaboration of state and federal agencies along with the private sector (Moynihan). The fire service was involved in the END emergency because its members understood ICS and the scale of the emergency required a management structure capable of managing a network of agencies.

It is unlikely that any member of the fire service had anticipated collaborating with veterinarians on such a scale before the END

CHAPTER 4 — COLLABORATE

What do you believe is the most important single service a collaborative network could provide your community in order to prevent or mitigate a catastrophe?

___ Information Sharing

___ Identifying Targets

___ Gathering Strategic Intelligence

___ Analyzing Strategic Intelligence

___ Producing Intelligence Products

___ Selecting Priority Risks

___ Joint Training

___ Joint Exercises

___ Joint Development of Strategy and Plans

___ Other, please specify: _____

_____

outbreak. Yet, for the current discussion, the important point to remember about ICS is that it occurs after an incident, rather than before an incident. Collaborating for prevention is a proactive communication and planning process occurring before an incident, aiming to preempt its occurrence or mitigate consequences ahead of the incident's occurrence. Therefore, prior incident management experiences and the agencies collaborating in responding to them do not determine the types of collaborative partners needed in preventing catastrophic harm to a community.

Partners can come from any number of areas. They may be public sector, private sector, non-profit, or community based.

The **public sector** is probably the most obvious choice for new alliances. In recent years, a general shift has occurred in government that encourages deal-making and partnering to deliver services more effectively. Collaboration is no exception. For example, there may be inroads to other jurisdictions or agencies through already established relationships or contractual agreements. There may be opportunities in prevention that have gone unnoticed and merit a second look.

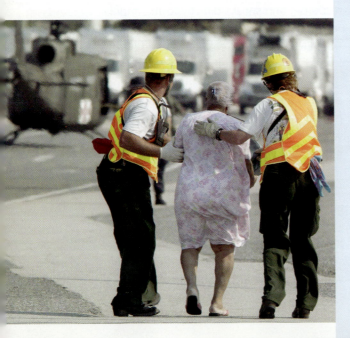

LEFT: *An elderly evacuee from New Orleans aided by Illinois State Forestry Service personnel from Southern Area Red Team. Joint Task Force effort in response to hurricane Katrina; September 2, 2005. Source: DefenseLINK.com, photo by MSGT Michael E. Best, USAF*

Potential partners in the local and regional public sector could range from utilities to Department of Defense assets. Identifying potential threats in the area might help determine which local agencies could be most helpful as strategic partners.

The **private sector** can bring a lot to the table. For example, recent reports indicate terrorists may plan to hijack trucks with hazardous materials for use in attacks. Local companies may have GPS tracking equipment that would help locate the vehicle. Without a preexisting relationship with the firm, getting access to the tracking data would be difficult and time consuming. The private sector has data-mining capabilities that can analyze trends. Government agencies may not be able to afford these tools let alone learn to use them in a timely manner.

Potential private partners are businesses in any industry that terrorists can use in an attack or suffer attack themselves. As with public partners, identifying potential threats helps in your selection of strategic private partners.

Many **community groups** should be included as well. For example, Firewise Communities promotes the National Wildland/Urban Interface Fire Program. The Wildland/Urban Interface Working Team (WUIWT) of the National Wildfire Coordinating Group directs and sponsors a consortium of wildland fire organizations and federal agencies responsible for wildland fire management in the United States. Programs such as "Got Clearance?" promote Firewise landscaping by occupancy owners living in areas susceptible to wildfires. Firewise landscaping reduces the wildfire threat to occupancies and involves collaboration between the Forest Service and local hardware stores and landscapers. (Agner) See the CD for more information about Firewise programs.

Additionally, the Community Emergency Response Team (CERT) program provides the fire service with opportunities to engage the community and build trusting relationships, while improving preparedness through training in basic disaster response skills. Each of these instances of engagement with the public provides an opportunity for information gathering and exchange with the community, a basic practice in the prevention of catastrophe.

At the national level, the U.S. Fire Administration provides a range of outreach programs to the community including the Preparedness Network (PrepNet), that delivers a distance learning and information system used by the United States Fire Administration (USFA) and other government agencies to virtually any community nationwide. USFA also provides many resources to the public on fire safety, as well as a range of courses for fire service professionals at the National Fire Academy. Links to these online resources are available on the CD.

Non-profit organizations can make helpful strategic partners. They are in touch with the community at the individual level and are effective at conducting public awareness and outreach programs. Government agencies are often ill equipped to handle complicated social issues such as drug abuse, infant mortality rates, and teen pregnancy. Non-profits excel in these areas and can bring similar results in building a prevention mindset among citizens. Potential partners include church groups, ethnic culture centers, and humanitarian agencies.

Approach collaboration as a process of building relationships with people involved in different activities than your own. Those collaborative partners can access distinct sources of information you may need in the future. In building a collaborative network, you need to communicate with people you ordinarily would not. To develop a collaborative relationship you must show up, perhaps by arranging a meeting at their office or other venue like a public event. Remain approachable and responsive, taking time to listen to the viewpoints of others, and learn from the differences and similarities with your own practices. The public considers the fire service among the easiest first responders to approach, so use that trust offered by the public in your profession to enhance your collaborative efforts.

There are many potential partners. Try to focus on those whose assistance you need—and those that are ready to contribute.

> Which entities do you expect will be easiest with which to collaborate? Why?

> Which entities do you expect will be most difficult with which to collaborate? Why?

Coleman Collaboration Equation

David Coleman has suggested **four criteria** to examine in **determining the readiness of an organization to collaborate:**

- **TECHNOLOGY:** Do you have the basic tools needed to collaborate?

- **CULTURE:** Do you have the attitudes and habits needed to make collaboration work?

- **ECONOMICS:** Is there a financial benefit to collaborating or financial disincentive for not collaborating?

- **POLITICS:** Does leadership and senior management believe in collaboration and practice what they say they believe? This can have a big impact on the other three criteria.

You may be ready to collaborate. You may want to collaborate. You may need to collaborate. Yet, unless your potential partner has similar needs and readiness, investment in collaboration is probably misplaced. **Coleman's equation is not a silver bullet.** Just because an organization scores high on its criteria doesn't mean it is necessarily a good partner for collaboration. Rather, the Coleman Equation provides a useful rule of thumb for thinking about the characteristics of prospective collaboration partners.

COLEMAN COLLABORATION EQUATION

$$\frac{\text{Technology} + (2 \times \text{Culture}) + (3 \times \text{Economics}) + (4 \times \text{Politics})}{\textit{Potential for Collaboration Success}}$$

Based on what you currently understand regarding your local community's most serious threats, vulnerabilities, and consequences, what do you believe are the **three most important candidates for collaboration?**

1 _____

2 _____

3 _____

Do you know enough about these candidates to assess if they are ready to collaborate with your local fire service agency?

    yes   no

Do you believe your fire service agency is ready to effectively collaborate?

    yes   no

CHAPTER 4 — COLLABORATE

Apply the Coleman Collaboration Equation.

Rate the organization 1 to 10 based on each factor. Be as honest as you can, and use the following scale.
A passing score is 80 or above.

	Technology	Culture	Economics	Politics	Totals
Your Organization					
Collaboration Candidate 1					
Collaboration Candidate 2					
Collaboration Candidate 3					

SCALE:

Technology = n
- 1 = Hard to find a computer in the enterprise.
- 10 = Employees can't live without e-mail, cell phones and other devices; T1 line to every desktop; high usage of Internet and intranet.

Culture x 2 = n
- 1 = Employees are asked to do their jobs, keep their heads down and their noses to the grindstone, and not pay attention to anyone else. The boss solves all problems and mandates actions.
- 10 = People routinely talk about important issues, much like a functional family around the dinner table; they work together as a team to solve problems.

Economics x 3 = n
- 1 = Collaboration will make no big operational difference to the agency nor will it affect the availability of fiscal resources.
- 10 = Collaboration is necessary for the effective use of fiscal resources.

Politics x 4 = n
- 1 = Talk about collaboration but don't do anything about it.
- 10 = Reaction of management: "We need it, we support and we will set the example by modeling collaborative behavior and using the tools."

SCORING:

Plug each factor's score into the box above and multiply by its weight for a subtotal. Then add them up for a total.

Scores below 60 are poor; 61 to 80 are fair. Scores above 80 are good and indicate a greater likelihood of collaborative success, or the possibility that your organization is already using collaborative tools successfully.

(The Coleman Collaboration Equation was developed by David Coleman and originally published in *CIO Magazine*.)

CHAPTER 4 — COLLABORATE

🏠 What kind of behavior do you personally find **trustworthy**?

_____
_____
_____
_____
_____
_____

What kind of behavior causes you to suspect someone is not trustworthy?

_____
_____
_____
_____
_____

If your fire service agency was a person would you trust him or her?

   yes   no

Why or why not?

_____
_____
_____
_____
_____
_____

UPPER RIGHT: *Collaboration is strong between Bloomington, Illinois Fire and Police Departments.*

Maintaining a Network

"Strategic partnering and alliancing is a process, not an event; a journey, not a destination." (*The Strategic Partnering Handbook*)

As this comment by Tony Lendrum suggests, creating a collaborative network is not a one-time task, but one that may be repeated many times. Once the network is going, it requires maintenance and refinements to continue working towards the collaborative goals.

Some important **aspects to consider in maintaining collaboration** include:

- **Build and maintain trust.**
- **Establish communication channels.**
- **Coordinate activities.**
- **Accommodate cultural differences.**

Each element is crucial to successful collaboration.

Trust is the cornerstone of collaboration.

Without trust, partners will be less likely to share information or cooperate. Gaining trust can be difficult. Some of the obstacles to overcome include rivalries, lack of incentives, organizational stovepipes, arrogant personalities, and untrustworthy behavior. Each one will require a solution specific to the circumstances. Fundamental to building trust is shared attention to mutual needs and mutual benefits.

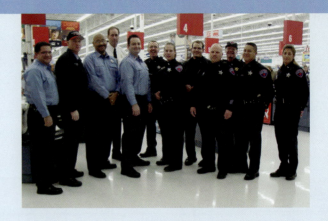

Establishing communication channels is also key to maintaining the network. Without it the network will quickly disappear. How often do you communicate? With whom? About what? Using what protocols? How do you share information? When do you choose not to share information?

Cultural difference is another area that will require attention in the collaborative network. Many groups may not be prepared to work together. For instance, non-profit groups tend to be humanitarian-focused while private sector businesses are more profit-focused.

Managing all of these elements will provide an outcome where **the whole of the relationships is greater than the sum of the parts**. A well-established network becomes easy to maintain because it is so clearly in everyone's mutual benefit to contribute to the network.

COLLABORATION AND SHARING INFORMATION

Information sharing and collaboration go hand in hand. Without collaboration there will not be much information sharing. Information sharing is usually the first step toward collaboration.

You cannot work together to solve a problem until you have begun to share information and analysis regarding the problem.

When one person or agency decides to take the risk of sharing information with another person or agency, they initiate the potential for collaboration.

A risk always exists that the information is misunderstood or misused and the source of the information takes the blame. The opportunity is that information gathered by one agency gives context to information gathered by another agency and provides both agencies a better understanding of reality.

If the receiving agency finds the information helpful and treats the source of information with respect, a seed of collaboration has been planted. If the receiving agency returns the favor and shares other information, another seed is planted. When one or both, or many, agencies begin to use the shared information, the seeds begin to sprout. Recognizing mutual benefit in sharing the information is like sunlight and water.

Deciding to establish regular channels and methods for sharing information is the difference between throwing seed on unprepared ground and carefully planting the seed in a cultivated garden. Collaboration significantly improves the likelihood of a good harvest: prevention of natural, accidental, and intentional catastrophe.

In Chapter 3, we noted that there are important sources of data and information that are probably easier for fire service agencies to gather. One agency cannot gather all the strategic (much less tactical) intelligence and interpret it for every locality. **A core concept of the prevention cube is to share the load for prevention** so that important information and the ability to act are not limited to a few.

Many first responder agencies currently view the creation of a strategic intelligence function as "too hard." Acting alone this is probably an accurate judgment. The potentially catastrophic outcome of not having a strategic intelligence function is also pretty tough. Purposeful collaboration is a way for your community to benefit from gathering, analyzing, and sharing strategic intelligence without any single agency paying the full cost.

Deciding to establish regular channels and methods for sharing information is the difference between throwing seed on unprepared ground and carefully planting the seed in a cultivated garden.

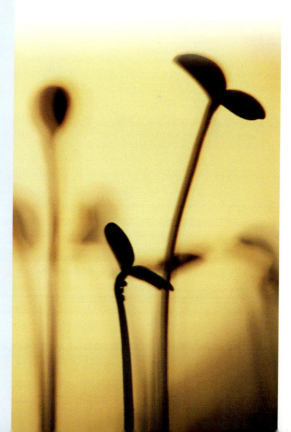

CHAPTER 4 — COLLABORATE

To develop a reasonably complete strategic picture for your community you need the following information:

❏ Identify specific natural threats:
_____
_____
_____

❏ Identify the capabilities of these natural threats:
_____
_____
_____

❏ Identify specific accidental threats:
_____
_____
_____

❏ Identify the capabilities of these accidental threats:
_____
_____
_____

❏ Identify specific intentional threats:
_____
_____
_____

❏ Identify the capabilities of these intentional threats:
_____
_____
_____

❏ Identify current specific vulnerabilities for each of the following sectors:

- Agricultural Sector
_____

- Banking and Financial System
_____

- Civic and Social Institutions (including public symbols)
_____

- Commercial/Industrial Facilities
_____

- Electric Power System
_____

- Emergency Services
_____

- Government Services
_____

- Information/Communications (including telecommunications and computers)
_____

- Public Health
_____

- Recreational Facilities
_____

- Transportation Centers
_____

- Water Supply
_____

- Other, please specify: _____

Information Needs

The most important information to share is what will allow you to answer the risk formula. What are your community's threats? What are your vulnerabilities? What are the potential consequences? You need help answering these questions. With the answers in hand you can make good decisions.

Likelihood x Consequences = Risk

$$\text{Likelihood} = \text{Threat} \begin{cases} \times \textbf{ Vulnerability if } \text{(state conditions)} \\ /\textbf{ Vulnerability if } \text{(state conditions)} \end{cases}$$

There are several potential "**offenders**" whether we are discussing natural, accidental or intentional threats. What are these threats? What are their capabilities? Do they have "**handlers**"? Sources of accidental threat certainly have handlers. Some would argue that terrorists have handlers. If so, can you collaborate in any way with the handlers? If you think in terms of threat capabilities, rather than specific threats, third-party handlers can affect a specific threat's offensive potential.

Each of the critical sectors listed at left might be considered the place where a specific target exists. How accessible are these places? Can you change the accessibility? Can you increase the deterrent effect? Can you improve protection? Who are the **managers** of these places? The managers are potentially important collaborators.

In the critical sectors there are specific **targets**. For example, in the water supply "place" there are sources, wellheads, purification systems, pipelines, distribution nodes, sewage lines, sewage treatment facilities and more. Who are the **guardians** of these targets? Such guardians are potentially important collaborators.

Without the cooperation of these potential collaborators you cannot gather the information you need to develop an accurate strategic picture. You need the collaboration of many others simply to gather the basic information. As you can probably already anticipate—and as we will examine carefully in the chapter on Managing Risk—you also need collaborators to effectively analyze the information.

Source: iStockphoto

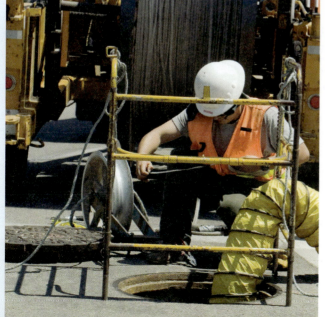

Organize the information utilizing the Routine Activity Theory (RAT) framework. This is sometimes also called the Problem Analysis Triangle (PAT).

[Triangle diagram: outer green triangle labeled Handler, Manager, Guardian; inner red triangle labeled Offender, Place, Target/Victim; center labeled CATASTROPHE]

 In terms of natural, accidental, or intentional catastrophe, what are the most vulnerable **"places"** in your community?

1

2

3

Who are the **"managers"** of these places?

1

2

3

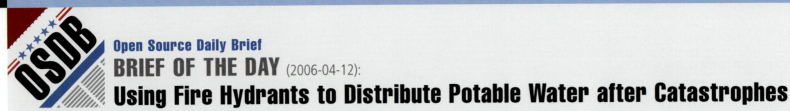

Open Source Daily Brief
BRIEF OF THE DAY (2006-04-12):
Using Fire Hydrants to Distribute Potable Water after Catastrophes

On the eve of the centennial of the Great Quake of 1906, San Francisco officials developed a new emergency resource from existing public utilities. Specifically, the program provides emergency drinking water from existing fire hydrants across the city.

Under the new program, the city is painting a blue water drop on water hydrants connected to major water mains throughout the city to signify their designation as hydrants suitable for emergency drinking water. These specific hydrants are on lines connected to reinforced water mains that can withstand moderate earthquakes.

If the city were to experience a major earthquake, emergency teams could tap the marked hydrants and distribute water to city residents from hydrants supplied with drinking water. Unmarked hydrants hold untreated water suitable only for use by firefighters. A spokesman for the San Francisco Public Utilities Commission, Tony Winnicker, says "[t]his plan is to mitigate some of the worst effects of a quake, so we don't face a New Orleans-like situation."

According to Winnicker, San Francisco has a week's supply of treated water stored in reservoirs and, if rationed, could stretch to weeks. However, he still cautions the public to take personal responsibility for preparedness by encouraging city residents "to store at least three days worth of water to use in the event of a quake."

The plan, developed with significant input from the San Francisco Police Department, Fire Department, and Office of Emergency Services, specifically addresses the procurement, transportation, and distribution of emergency drinking water to the public.

"The San Francisco Fire Department and the SFPUC worked closely to develop this plan and ensure that after a major earthquake or disaster, we can accomplish the twin priorities of fighting fires and providing emergency drinking water," said SFFD Chief Joanne Hayes-White.

The San Francisco Public Utilities Commission publicized the emergency drinking water campaign at community events by handing out brochures with maps highlighting the 67 hydrants' locations.

PREVENTION RELEVANCE: Issue-specific preparedness used to mitigate catastrophic situations is a tool of prevention.

PREVENTION TECHNIQUES: Collaborate with other public agencies and private enterprises to establish an emergency drinking water plan. Inspect and reinforce water lines, as needed, while identifying and clearly marking hydrants connected to suitable drinking water supplies.

PREVENTION THOUGHT: Potable water is an essential element of any preparedness plan. Can you think of circumstances where it is better to treat and store drinking water than use a hydrant plan?

The Open Source Daily Brief is a service of the Institute for Preventive Strategies (©IPS). You can register to receive the OSDBs at www.preventivestrategies.net.

COLLABORATION AND IDENTIFYING TARGETS

In the first chapter of this workbook, we asked you to use your imagination to identify potential targets. Many of the potential collaborators we identified possess significant existing expertise regarding their "places" and "targets." They also need to use their imagination, but their imagination has much more detailed knowledge on which to draw.

You obviously have to start with your own understanding of the threat. This understanding will help you identify important potential collaborators.

As you begin to work together with these collaborators your perception of the threat is likely to shift. It will probably expand. This is good. This means you are less likely to ignore a potential threat or vulnerability. Through sharing information and working together on target identification, your community can better prepare for any natural, accidental, or intentional threat.

Our terrorist adversaries mostly organize themselves as a collaborative network. This structure is flexible, resilient, and can span significant scope and scale with modest resources. We can play the same game and almost certainly play it better.

One of the first collaboration-building or information-sharing activities you might want to host is a target and vulnerability identification workshop. Just getting together to create this list will begin to make the introductions, communicate the purpose, and build the social capital that can lead to more information sharing and ongoing collaboration.

REGIONAL COLLABORATION

Prevention and mitigation of catastrophe is almost by definition a regional responsibility. If a disaster is localized—limited to a defined space—and can be effectively managed with only local resources then it is probably not a catastrophe.

A catastrophe quickly overwhelms local resources and directly affects more than one jurisdiction. If you are giving priority to catastrophic threats then collaboration across your region is a practical requirement.

In many cases, the Department of Homeland Security already requires formal regional planning as a condition of receiving grants. For example, DHS grant guidance for the Urban Area Security Initiative (UASI) states:

> In updating their homeland security strategies, States and Urban Areas are asked to examine current regional collaboration efforts and explore new approaches to developing regional capabilities. The strategy should provide a narrative description of how the State

---

In terms of natural, accidental, or intentional catastrophe, what/who are the most likely **"victims"** in your community?

1 _____

2 _____

3 _____

Who are the **"guardians"** of these victims?

1 _____

2 _____

3 _____

Did you consider the elderly, seriously ill, and very poor?

_____
_____

Are guardians sometimes absent?

_____
_____

CHAPTER 4 — COLLABORATE

🏠 Are there any preexisting organizations that involve many of the managers of the vulnerable places you identified?

_____
_____
_____
_____
_____
_____
_____
_____
_____

Are there any preexisting organizations that involve many of the guardians of the potential victims you identified?

_____
_____
_____
_____
_____
_____
_____
_____
_____

or Urban Area currently uses and plans to use mutual aid to prevent, protect against, respond to, and recover from major events. The strategy should present the States' or Urban Areas' vision for increasing existing collaboration efforts.... In developing this vision and updating their strategies, States and Urban Areas should complete the following activities:

- Define current collaboration efforts already undertaken across jurisdictions and across disciplines within jurisdictions

- Discuss opportunities for future collaboration with other geographic regions that can enhance capability within the State or Urban Area

- Define future goals and objectives for a regional approach for prevention, protection, response, and recovery

- Outline a process for integrating operational systems from multiple disciplines and jurisdictions for all mission areas

It is important to note that regional collaboration is not necessarily a structured, institutionalized program across regions, but better defined as a strategic vision for the future, with a multi-jurisdictional and multi-disciplinary approach to homeland security.

There is not a one-size-fits-all approach to regional collaboration, but the States' or Urban Areas' vision should support an enterprise-wide approach to building capability for all the mission areas.

Hurricane Katrina—and most hurricanes—demonstrate that serious natural disasters are regional issues, not just local issues. If pandemic influenza is to be contained, it will require a very rapid local response that is closely coordinated on a regional basis.

The regional scope of an accidental threat is generally much smaller than a natural disaster, but it may still span multiple jurisdictions, often encompassing several cities and more than one county. When, as is often the case, a major urban area spans more than one state, regional collaboration is especially difficult to organize.

If terrorists choose to deploy weapons of catastrophe, the impact area will almost certainly cover a hundred square miles or more, compared to the one square mile most seriously affected by 9/11.

CHAPTER 4 — COLLABORATE

As the Fire Chief for the fictional City of San Luis Rey which of the "regions" shown on the map do you consider most important for your catastrophe prevention effort?

What criteria did you use in making your choice?

San Luis Rey® is a fictional jurisdiction designed by Teleologic Learning LLC. All characters, locations, and events are fictitious and intended for instructional purposes only.

Does your fire service agency currently participate in any mutual aid agreements?

yes   no   I don't know

If yes, with what entities?

_____
_____
_____
_____
_____
_____

For what purposes?

_____
_____
_____
_____
_____
_____

COLLABORATIVE AGREEMENTS

If well-organized collaboration is like a good garden, then some communities and regions will decide to try full-blown farming.

Consider the urban firestorms that consumed Chicago in 1871 and threatened Boston in 1872. The Fire Chief in Boston, John Damrell, had visited Chicago and learned what he could from the fire there. He quickly recognized the severity of the Boston fire that broke out in November 1872. The City of Boston had state-of-the-art pumping equipment and well-trained firefighters. However, Damrell faced a situation in which all the workhorses were down with equestrian distemper and too sick to leave their stalls, requiring the firefighters to draw the fire pumps along cobblestone streets. Also, the height of the buildings in downtown Boston meant that the fire jumped from building to building since the pumps' water pressure was not sufficient to reach the tops of the buildings.

Damrell realized the situation was primed to replicate the devastation of the Chicago fire a year earlier. He sent a request to all fire departments within fifty miles of Boston, the first call for mutual aid in fire service history. Firefighters from as far away as New Haven, Connecticut and Biddeford, Maine showed up nine hours after Damrell sent out his call. As a result, the "Great Boston Fire of 1872 became the first urban firestorm ever to be successfully contained" (Flynn, Stephen).

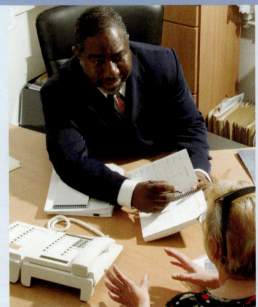

Collaboration can take many forms:

INFORMAL: In many cases, this is sufficient—even better—than other methods. Getting to know your peers in other Preparedness Professions, sharing notes, meeting for coffee, understanding each other's roles, and building trust over time contributes a great deal to the prevention and mitigation of catastrophe.

FACILITATED: In some cases—especially in larger jurisdictions and across a region—there is the need to host regular meetings, share e-mail and phone lists, conduct joint training, and make a regular effort to build social capital, share information, identify targets, and over time craft a truly collaborative relationship.

FORMAL: Whether your community starts with informal connections or something more ambitious, as individuals and agencies become comfortable with collaboration they often recognize the benefit of formalizing collaborative channels.

In the past, formal agreements tended to focus on mutual aid in response to disaster. There is an increasing trend—encouraged by federal dollars and regulation—to move toward formal agreements related to joint planning, training, and the operation of multi-jurisdictional Incident Command Systems.

The National Emergency Management Association has developed a Model Intrastate Mutual Aid Legislation (see the CD) that encourages jurisdictions to shift focus from response to all aspects of preparedness including prevention of catastrophes. According to the model legislation:

> The system shall provide for mutual assistance among the participating political subdivisions in the prevention of, response to, and recovery from, any disaster that results in a formal state of emergency in a participating political subdivision, subject to that participating political subdivision's criteria for declaration. The system shall provide for mutual cooperation among the participating subdivisions in conducting disaster related exercises, testing or other training activities outside actual declared emergency periods.

Most formal collaborative agreements are frameworks without detailed operational specifications. The frameworks cover how a jurisdiction joins or declines to join an agreement, when to make an agreement operational, how financial issues are handled, and how to minimize issues of legal liability. Otherwise, there is a need for collaborative agencies to decide how they will actually work together.

In working together to prevent catastrophe, there will be a healthy level of trial-and-error in developing standard operating procedures for intergovernmental, multi-agency, and public-private collaboration. However, if you begin the collaborative process with information sharing, and then involve the key parties in truly joint threat recognition, you will have a strong foundation for moving forward in other ways.

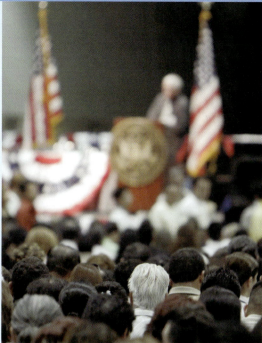

Source: iStockphoto

Collaboration often does not work. In your experience, what is the biggest **impediment** to effective collaboration?

____ Lack of mutual self-interest

____ Lack of time and opportunity to develop habits of collaboration

____ Poor leadership

____ Competition in funding

____ Untrustworthy behavior

____ Insufficient joint training and/or exercising

____ Other, please specify: _____

____ Other, please specify: _____

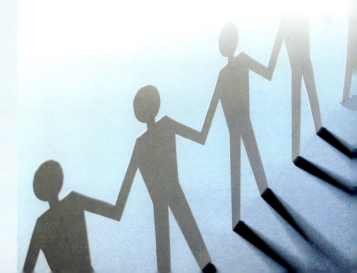

COLLABORATE:
Chapter Review

What is another way to say you are collaborating?

What is the Coleman Collaboration Equation?

What is the benefit of collaboration for information sharing?

You collaborate within a network of partners. What differentiates a circle of friends from collaboration?

What is the most important, most heavily weighted, factor in the Coleman Collaboration Equation?

What is the benefit of collaboration for target identification?

What criteria should you apply to selecting members of your collaborative network?

For what purpose can you use the Coleman Collaboration Equation?

CHAPTER 4 — COLLABORATE

APPLY WHAT YOU HAVE LEARNED

🔘 **Use your CD to access the Collaboration Advanced Exercise.** Select the **Chapter 4** Certificate Course link located in the Online Exercises section of your CD.

Collaboration is the cornerstone to preventing catastrophe. *It is now 18 months before a planned terrorist attack.* **Your collaboration network has alerted you to a new potential threat in San Luis Rey®. The situation is changing.** Is your collaboration network sufficiently broad and flexible to provide you with the information you will need to assess this threat?

Using the principles of this workbook you will be challenged to develop a strategic collaborative network that is able to provide information, consultation, and guidance on the emerging terrorist threat.

Senior Fire Department Captains state their collaboration network strategies and choices. Can you accurately assess their collaboration plan's strengths and weaknesses?

Note: If you have already enrolled in the Homeland Security Terrorism Prevention Certificate Course for Fire Service Professionals (©IPS) you can go directly to the exercise by using the Online Exercises Direct Access links on your CD or by typing this URL into your browser's address window:

www.preventivestrategies.net/go/ mhfs-adv-ex-collaborate

For first time access, use this initial URL:
www.preventivestrategies.net/go/ mhfs-enroll

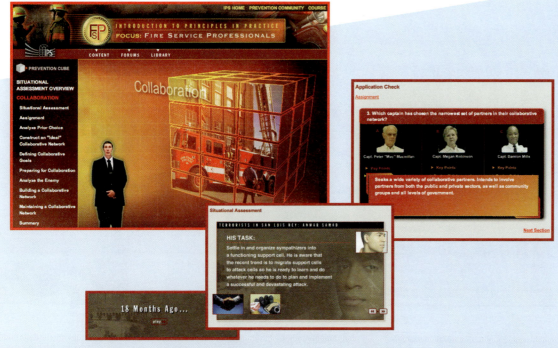
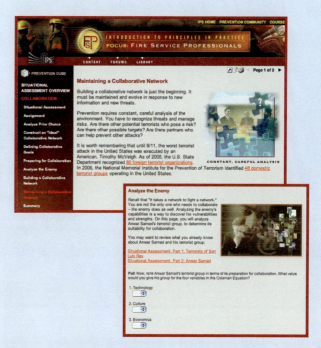

San Luis Rey® is a fictional jurisdiction designed by Teleologic Learning LLC.
All characters, locations, and events are fictitious and intended for instructional purposes only.

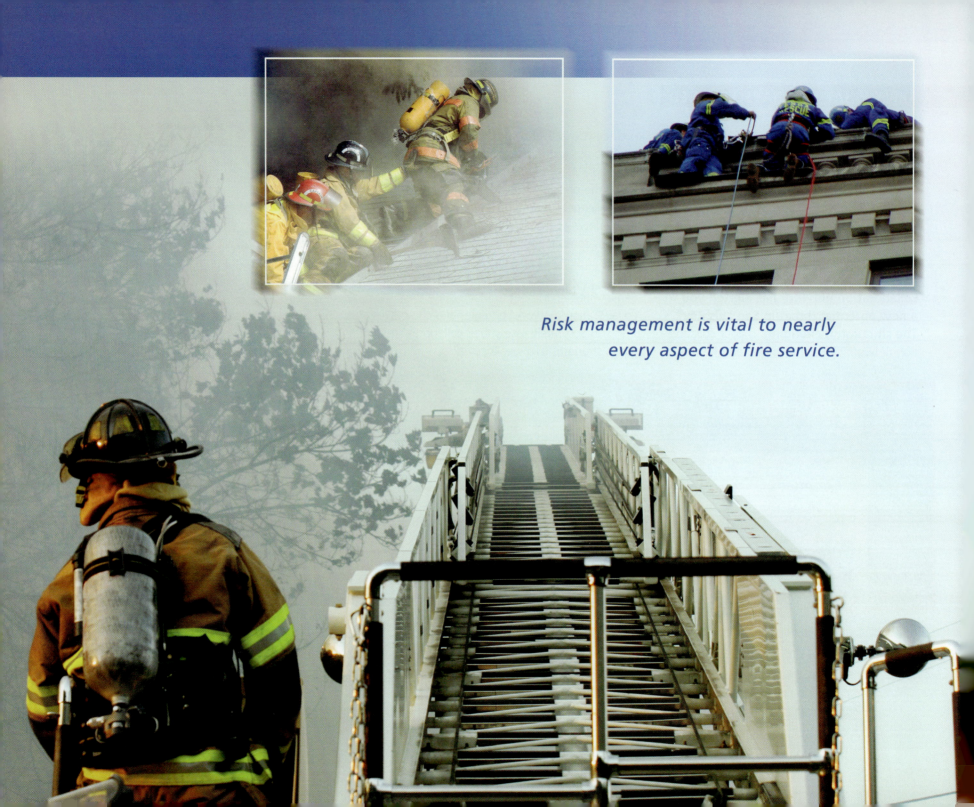

Risk management is vital to nearly every aspect of fire service.

Manage Risk

✓ *In this chapter you will learn:*
- How current priorities influence your ability to manage risk.
- How you make risk management choices every day.
- How to focus on the most consequential risk.
- How to use scenarios to think through your community's risk.
- How to collaborate without just compromising.
- How to manage risk by transfer, avoidance, reduction, or acceptance.
- How to continually assess risk management choices.

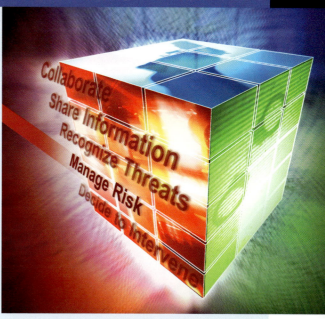

*You cannot do everything, so you must decide what you reasonably **can** do.*

The fire service focuses a great deal of attention on the risk to personal safety that its members face while responding to incidents. How to carry an axe or Halligan tool safely, lift a ladder, breech a door, look for signs of an impending backdraft, pull a ceiling, or trench a roof, etc. is drilled into firefighters from day one. Just about every action a firefighter takes at an emergency incident carries with it risk and danger. Yet, risk management for the fire service goes well beyond concerns for individual safety. In fact, risk management in the fire service is a vital element entwined with nearly every aspect of the work (Stewart).

In this chapter, you will learn to use the principles of the prevention cube to approach the challenge of managing the risks associated with the fire service role in preparing for, and preventing, catastrophic events. There are several basic steps. First, you choose partners and develop effective ways to collaborate. After choosing collaboration partners, you need to gather, evaluate, and analyze strategic information from a number of sources. You will share information among the collaborative partners. Together you will identify a whole range of natural, accidental, and intentional threats.

Once you have done this, it is time to make some tough choices. Making tough choices usually presents serious challenges to collaboration. As a group, you need to consider the potential threats, vulnerabilities, and consequences to decide which poses the most catastrophic consequences to your community. Which risks do you treat as the highest priority? Which should receive continuous attention? Given your resources—time, personnel, money, and more—how will you limit your choices? Choosing which risks to assign priority attention is often a source of serious disagreement. Yet, without a clear choice that preparedness professions will genuinely support, your community cannot successfully prevent or mitigate catastrophe.

Identifying and prioritizing risks is about accepting tradeoffs. You cannot do everything, so you must decide what you reasonably can do. As new information emerges, you must be flexible about adjusting priorities. However, in all cases, you must keep your priorities clear.

FACING PAGE: *Background: iStockphoto. Inset Left: Bloomington, IL Fire Department. Inset Right: Sangamon County Rescue Squad, photo by Jerry McKay*

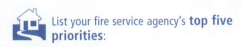

List your fire service agency's **top five priorities**:

1 _____

2 _____

3 _____

4 _____

5 _____

Who set these priorities?

_____
_____
_____

CURRENT PRIORITIES

What are the current priorities of your fire service agency? Are these priorities clear and understood by all? Are any of the priorities informal and not always observed? Sometimes priorities remain largely unspoken or informal and still prove effective. If this is the case with your agency, how do members recognize those largely unspoken priorities? How are they chosen? Who makes the choice? How is attention to priorities encouraged and reinforced?

Do any of the current priorities relate to preventing catastrophe or preparing for disaster? Are you aware of the priorities chosen by other preparedness professions in your area? Is there any overlap in the current priorities of police, emergency management, public health, fire safety and others?

Given current priorities, what attitudes exist in your community about preventing catastrophe? Answers differ widely from place to place. In many Florida communities, for example, the ongoing risk of hurricanes may have resulted in policies, procedures, and protocols that are adaptable to other catastrophic threats. On the other hand, even communities with known vulnerabilities can go for a long time without experiencing a catastrophe or 'near miss.' In this case, it may be more difficult to motivate people to keep in mind the potential for catastrophe.

APPLY A RISK FORMULA

Consider the idea that

Risk = Likelihood x Consequences.

Is the greater risk one that is more likely, or one that has more severe consequences? You are more likely to catch a winter cold than have a heart attack. But, which is the *greater* risk, a winter cold or a heart attack?

You may very well want to take action to reduce both the risk of a winter cold and a heart attack. You may take a multi-vitamin and regularly wash your hands to avoid a cold. You may watch your diet and regularly exercise to avoid a heart attack. How does your perception of future risk influence your behavior now? Do you act intentionally to prevent risk?

When you buy health insurance, which risk is more on your mind, the winter cold or the heart attack? Is health insurance an example of prevention, response, or recovery?

If you had a cold would you see a physician or go to bed, self-medicate, and drink plenty of fluids? Maybe you would go to work and share the cold with co-workers. If you felt a sudden sharp pain in your left shoulder, what would you do?

When considering these situations and responses you are engaging in risk management. You are evaluating risk based on your personal attitudes and knowledge of likelihood and consequences.

Most people are unaware of the process they use to make these decisions. They tend not to think about future risks. The same people who buy health insurance to manage the consequences of illness may not invest in simple preventive care, such as hand-washing or eating healthy foods, unless the perceived risk is very real.

The son of a man who died young of a heart attack is usually more attentive to heart care. A person with a weak immune system will be more concerned about the threat of a cold. If we feel vulnerable to a threat, that threat seems more likely. Recognition of the likelihood increases our attention to the threat.

Likelihood x Consequences = Risk

Likelihood = Threat $\begin{cases} \times \textbf{\textit{Vulnerability if}} \text{ (state conditions)} \\ / \textbf{\textit{Vulnerability if}} \text{ (state conditions)} \end{cases}$

For the most part though, our attention to a catastrophic health event centers on managing consequences rather than preventing the event itself. There is an element of time that helps to explain this inconsistency. If the threat seems distant and the vulnerability is unclear, we often **make choices that actually increase our risk**.

Risk management involves well-defined current costs that have ill-defined future payoffs.

Preventing the 'common' cold we may never get requires an investment of time and money. We may have to buy a multi-vitamin, spend 10 seconds every morning to take the vitamin and, maybe, three minutes each day to wash our hands. Rationally this is a small price to pay to significantly reduce our risk. Getting a good night's sleep is a simple and effective preventive measure. But some people are not willing to 'spend' their time in this way. Part of the problem is that even if we take all these preventive steps we may still catch a cold. We may reduce the risk, but we cannot eliminate the risk.

The personal costs of preventing a heart attack are higher still. We may need to cut back on some of our favorite foods, exercise several times a week, and even take some regular medications. These measures can help us avoid a much more serious consequence. Still, many of us won't pay the price. We know we should. We recognize the risk. But, we ignore the likelihood and the consequences. We may even choose a lifestyle that increases our vulnerability. Even after a heart attack **some victims continue to behave in a manner that increases vulnerability to the next attack**. Unless threat and vulnerability are very real we discount both. Even if the consequences are dire we can still deny the risk.

This is basically the same thinking and behavior we see in most of our communities. It is irrational. It also is typically human.

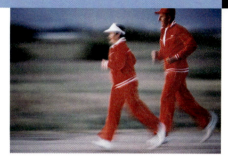

The same people who buy health insurance to manage the consequences of illness may not invest in simple preventive care.

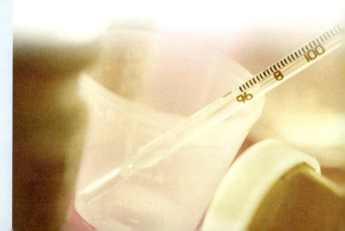

CHAPTER 5 — MANAGE RISK

In traditional fire service work, which data and information are scanned and analyzed?

_____
_____
_____
_____
_____
_____
_____

Is there any overlap in the data and information already scanned and analyzed and what you need to examine to prevent catastrophe?

_____
_____
_____
_____

If yes, how do you need to treat the same information? Should you distribute it differently?

_____
_____
_____
_____
_____
_____

SARA AND RISK MANAGEMENT

In your private life, you may be as irrational as anyone else. However, the fire service professional differs from his or her civilian counterparts in training, education, experience, and expertise in applying rational methods to the solution of problems.

In your work as a firefighter, you may have already been trained to **Scan, Analyze, Respond, and Assess (SARA)**. In many ways these same steps are key to managing risk.

SCAN: Sharing information is a way to scan. Identifying potential threats is another way to scan.

ANALYZE: When you begin to organize information and produce intelligence products you are engaged in analysis.

RESPOND: When you choose how to respond to your scanning and your analysis you are often practicing risk management. You are selecting what is most important from what you have scanned. You are using analysis to inform this choice.

ASSESS: In this stage you review and evaluate the first three steps. You evaluate your response for effectiveness.

The intelligence products outlined in the previous chapter on Sharing Information can be very important to this process. They are a way to organize data from scanning and analyzing. And, they will help to focus your response.

But no matter how rigorous your analysis, you will rarely find a single right way to manage the problem. You will almost always be faced with a range of potential responses. **Your optimal response will:**

1. **Depend on available resources.**
2. **Prove effective depending on the nature of the risk.**
3. **Focus on the most consequential risk.**

Selecting the risk that is most consequential is a key decision in risk management. Trying to prevent a heart attack is more important than trying to prevent a winter cold. But with risk management the choice is seldom that easy. It is more likely that your scanning and analyzing will expose several problems and many risks.

CHOOSING AMONG RISKS

What are your community's vulnerabilities?

Where are you vulnerable?

Are you equally vulnerable to natural, accidental, and intentional threats? Or are you more vulnerable to certain kinds of threats?

Which combination of threat and vulnerability results in the most likely risk?

Which combination of threat and vulnerability results in the most catastrophic risk?

How can you reasonably assess your comparative risk?

There are many methods for evaluating threats and vulnerabilities. A helpful introduction to several models is available from the National Oceanic and Atmospheric Administration. (See link on the CD.)

One method is **to identify a group of experts** on your local vulnerabilities and another group on your local threats. **Develop questionnaires** that each of the experts complete anonymously. **Tabulate the results. Share the anonymous results** with the experts and seek clarification. Try to eventually **reduce the questionnaires to a numeric scale** that the experts use to assess each vulnerability and each threat.

The expert panel on vulnerabilities will probably include those with significant familiarity with your local economy, built environment, health care system, technical infrastructure, and other community assets. Their first job would be to assess which failures will create the greatest harm regardless of cause. Just as an example, suppose the vulnerability panel might produce a list of comparative vulnerabilities like the following:

Electrical Grid Failure — Vulnerability Level 9
Health System Failure — Vulnerability Level 7
Water Supply Failure — Vulnerability Level 10

Another group of experts could assess the different threats facing your community. This panel is likely to consist of public health professionals, police and intelligence officials, transportation officials, geologists, meteorologists and others familiar with natural, accidental, and intentional threats. This panel might identify what they consider the most serious threats. Just as an example, suppose this panel identifies a hurricane as the top threat facing your community. It would then be helpful to ask your vulnerability experts to reevaluate their assessments specifically in terms of a hurricane threat. In this way, you are using a systematic method for quantifying how your threats interact with your vulnerabilities. The result is an assessment of Likelihood.

Likelihood x *Consequences* = *Risk*

$$\text{Likelihood} = \text{Threat} \begin{cases} \times \text{ Vulnerability if (state conditions)} \\ / \text{ Vulnerability if (state conditions)} \end{cases}$$

Once you have completed these separate and anonymous procedures for determining Likelihood you could bring together your threat and vulnerability experts to consider the issue of consequences. Which threat interacting with which vulnerabilities produces the most serious consequences? Which will result in highest mortality, the greatest economic harm, the most long-term harm? Which interaction of threat and vulnerability

---

What are your community's **most significant** vulnerabilities?

What is the potential for a natural, accidental, or intentional threat to affect those vulnerabilities?

Answering these two questions will identify your most likely disasters.

Of those likely disasters, which poses the **most catastrophic consequences**?

has the most catastrophic consequences? The Department of Homeland Security's Asset-based Risk Analysis model includes human health, economic resources, strategic mission, and psychological outcomes as four key elements of consequence. Looking at each of these elements in the context of your most likely threats may be a good place to start.

Using anonymous questionnaires should minimize the "politics" involved in making choices. However, in contemplating consequences, there may be real benefit for experts to interact with each other, imagine worst-cases, and define some scenarios that will help define your local consequences. The definition of consequence is especially important given the influence that consequence has in defining risk.

Risk = Likelihood x Consequences

Likelihood can be managed by reducing threat or vulnerability. But the potential consequence is often more or less static. As a result, consequence has a powerful effect on how we define risk.

(Using expert panels as outlined above is sometimes called the Delphi Method. More information on this method can be found at http://www.is.njit.edu/pubs/delphibook/. The Delphi Method is often used by the Department of Homeland Security. Some find this method unreliable. A critique of the Delphi Method can be found at http://www.rand.org/pubs/reports/R1283/)

Your CD includes a reading that outlines other methods of Risk Management. Please access *Integrating Risk Management with Security and Antiterrorism Resource Allocation Decision Making* by Parnell, Dillon-Miller, and Bresnick.

SCENARIO-BASED RISK ASSESSMENT

Expert panels can help your community define risk. The Strategic Intelligence Products that emerge from the Sharing Information stage will help define your local risks. Even some simply structured discussion of potential threats can help highlight risks that are not yet receiving regular attention.

You can also use scenarios to facilitate "real world" consideration of comparative risk. According to Max Bazerman and Michael Watkins, "The goal of scenario planning is to help organizations identify and quantify risk, so that they neither take on unrecognized risk nor, critically, become overly risk averse." (*Predictable Surprises*)

The Department of Homeland Security has developed **fifteen planning scenarios** to assist your community and region develop a more thorough risk assessment. Following are the bare bones of each scenario as developed by DHS. A more complete description of all fifteen scenarios is provided on your CD.

Which of these scenarios do you perceive would be most helpful for your local community or region to use in risk assessment? (Use the space below to write your answers.)

For the purposes of risk assessment these fifteen scenarios should help communities:

- **Identify threat capabilities, regardless of the specific source.**
- **Identify the catastrophic potential of the threat capabilities.**
- **Identify potential critical vulnerabilities relevant to each scenario.**
- **Identify the key Preparedness Professions involved in prevention, response and recovery of each scenario.**

Which of the scenarios on pages 117-121 do you perceive would be most helpful for your local community or region to use in risk assessment? Select no more than three.

1 _____

2 _____

3 _____

15 NIGHTMARES FOR DISASTER PLANNING
—Adapted from planning scenarios developed by the U.S. Department of Homeland Security

Nuclear Detonation — 1
10-Kiloton Improvised Nuclear Device

CASUALTIES: can vary widely
INFRASTRUCTURE DAMAGE: total within radius of 0.5 to 1.0 mile
EVACUATIONS/DISPLACED PERSONS: 450,000 or more
CONTAMINATION: approx. 3,000 sq. miles
ECONOMIC IMPACT: hundreds of billions of dollars
POTENTIAL FOR MULTIPLE EVENTS: no
RECOVERY TIMELINE: years

SCENARIO OVERVIEW: In this scenario, terrorists assemble a gun-type nuclear device using highly enriched uranium (HEU) (used here to mean weapons-grade uranium) stolen from a nuclear facility located in the former Soviet Union. The nuclear device components are smuggled into the United States. The 10-kiloton nuclear device is assembled near a major metropolitan center. Using a delivery van, terrorists transport the device to the central business district of a large city and detonate it. Most buildings within 1,000 meters (~3,200 feet) of the detonation are severely damaged. Injuries from flying debris (missiles) may occur out to 6 kilometers (~ 3.7 miles). An Electro-magnetic Pulse (EMP) damages many electronic devices within about 5 kilometers (~ 3 miles). A mushroom cloud rises above the city and begins to drift north-east.

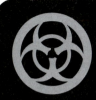

Biological Attack — 2
Aerosol Anthrax

CASUALTIES: 13,000 fatalities and injuries
INFRASTRUCTURE DAMAGE: minimal, other than contamination
EVACUATIONS/DISPLACED PERSONS: possibly
CONTAMINATION: extensive
ECONOMIC IMPACT: billions of dollars
POTENTIAL FOR MULTIPLE EVENTS: yes
RECOVERY TIMELINE: months

SCENARIO OVERVIEW: Anthrax spores delivered by aerosol result in inhalation anthrax, which develops when the bacterial organism, Bacillus anthracis, is inhaled into the lungs. A progressive infection follows. This scenario describes a single aerosol anthrax attack in one city delivered by a truck using a concealed improvised spraying device in a densely populated urban city with a significant commuter workforce. It does not, however, exclude the possibility of multiple attacks in disparate cities or time-phased attacks (i.e., "reload"). For federal planning purposes, it will be assumed that the Universal Adversary (UA) will attack five separate metropolitan areas in a sequential manner. Three cities will be attacked initially, followed by two additional cities 2 weeks later.

Biological Disease Outbreak — 3
Pandemic Influenza

CASUALTIES: at a 15% attack rate: 87,000 fatalities; 300,000 hospitalizations
INFRASTRUCTURE DAMAGE: none
EVACUATIONS/DISPLACED PERSONS: isolation of exposed persons
CONTAMINATION: none
ECONOMIC IMPACT: $70 to $160 billion
POTENTIAL FOR MULTIPLE EVENTS: yes, would be worldwide nearly simultaneously
RECOVERY TIMELINE: several months

SCENARIO OVERVIEW: Influenza pandemics have occurred every 10 to 60 years, with three occurring in the 20th century. Influenza pandemics occur when there is a notable genetic shift in the circulating strain of influenza. Because of this genetic shift, a large portion of the human population is entirely vulnerable to infection from the new pandemic strain. In this scenario twenty-five cases occur first in a small village in south China. Over the next 2 months, outbreaks begin to appear in Hong Kong, Singapore, South Korea, and Japan. Although cases are reported in all age groups, young adults appear to be the most severely affected, and case-fatality rates approach 5%. Several weeks later, the virus appears in four major U.S. cities. By nature, pandemic influenza moves extremely rapidly, and the outbreaks continue.

CHAPTER 5 — MANAGE RISK

Biological Attack 4
Plague

- **CASUALTIES:** 2,500 fatalities; 7,000 injuries
- **INFRASTRUCTURE DAMAGE:** none
- **EVACUATIONS/DISPLACED PERSONS:** possibly
- **CONTAMINATION:** lasts for hours
- **ECONOMIC IMPACT:** millions of dollars
- **POTENTIAL FOR MULTIPLE EVENTS:** no
- **RECOVERY TIMELINE:** years

SCENARIO OVERVIEW: Plague is a bacterium that causes high mortality in untreated cases and has epidemic potential. It is best known as the cause of Justinian's Plague (in the middle sixth century) and the Black Death (in the middle fourteenth century), two pandemics that killed millions. In this scenario, members of the Universal Adversary (UA) release pneumonic plague into three main areas of a major metropolitan city—in the bathrooms of the city's major airport, at the city's main sports arena, and at the city's major train station.

Chemical Attack 5
Blister Agent

- **CASUALTIES:** 150 fatalities; 70,000 hospitalized
- **INFRASTRUCTURE DAMAGE:** minimal
- **EVACUATIONS/DISPLACED PERSONS:** more than 100,000
- **CONTAMINATION:** structures affected
- **ECONOMIC IMPACT:** $500 million
- **POTENTIAL FOR MULTIPLE EVENTS:** yes
- **RECOVERY TIMELINE:** weeks; many long-term health affects

SCENARIO OVERVIEW: Agent YELLOW is a liquid mixture of sulfur Mustard and Lewisite with a garlic-like odor. Inhaling this mixture may cause respiratory damage while contact with skin or eyes can result in serious burns. High-level exposure can be fatal. In this scenario, the Universal Adversary (UA) uses a light aircraft to spray agent YELLOW into a college football stadium contaminating the stadium and the surrounding area and creating a downwind vapor hazard. The majority of casualties require urgent and long-term medical treatment. Few immediate fatalities occur. 70% of the stadium population is immediately exposed to the liquid. The remaining 30% (in the covered areas) plus 10% of the population in the vapor hazard area are exposed to vapor contamination.

Chemical Attack 6
Toxic Industrial Chemicals

- **CASUALTIES:** 350 fatalities; 1,000 hospitalizations
- **INFRASTRUCTURE DAMAGE:** 50% of structures in area of explosion
- **EVACUATIONS/DISPLACED PERSONS:** up to 700,000
- **CONTAMINATION:** yes
- **ECONOMIC IMPACT:** billions of dollars
- **POTENTIAL FOR MULTIPLE EVENTS:** yes
- **RECOVERY TIMELINE:** months

SCENARIO OVERVIEW: In this scenario, Universal Adversary (UA) terrorists land several helicopters at fixed facility petroleum refineries. They launch rocket-propelled grenades (RPGs) and plant improvised explosive devices (IEDs) before re-boarding and departing. The result is major fires and multiple cargo containers explode either aboard or near cargo ships. Two of the ships contain flammable liquids or solids. A north-northeast wind carries a large plume of smoke containing various metals into heavily populated areas. One of the burning ships contains resins and coatings including isocyanates, nitriles, and epoxy resins. Some IEDs are set for delayed detonation. Casualties occur onsite due to explosive blast and fragmentation, fire, and vapor or liquid exposure to the toxic industrial chemical (TIC). Downwind casualties occur due to vapor exposure.

CHAPTER 5 — MANAGE RISK

Chemical Attack 7

Nerve Agent

CASUALTIES: 6,000 fatalities (95% of building occupants); 350 injuries
INFRASTRUCTURE DAMAGE: minimal, other than contamination
EVACUATIONS/DISPLACED PERSONS: yes
CONTAMINATION: extensive
ECONOMIC IMPACT: $300 million
POTENTIAL FOR MULTIPLE EVENTS: extensive
RECOVERY TIMELINE: 3 to 4 months

SCENARIO OVERVIEW: Sarin is a human-made chemical warfare nerve agent. Nerve agents are the most toxic and rapidly acting of the known chemical warfare agents. A clear, colorless, and tasteless liquid that has no odor in its pure form, Sarin can evaporate into a vapor and spread into the environment. Sarin is also known as GB. In this scenario, the Universal Adversary (UA) builds six spray dissemination devices and releases Sarin vapor into the ventilation systems of three large commercial office buildings in a metropolitan area. The agent kills 95% of the people in the buildings and kills or sickens many of the first responders. In addition, some of the agent exits through rooftop ventilation stacks, creating a downwind hazard.

Chemical Attack 8

Chlorine Tank Explosion

CASUALTIES: 17,500 fatalities; 10,000 severe injuries; 100,000 hospitalizations
INFRASTRUCTURE DAMAGE: in immediate explosions areas, and metal corrosion in areas of heavy exposure
EVACUATIONS/DISPLACED PERSONS: up to 70,000 (self evacuate)
CONTAMINATION: primarily at explosion site, and if waterways are impacted
ECONOMIC IMPACT: millions of dollars
POTENTIAL FOR MULTIPLE EVENTS: yes
RECOVERY TIMELINE: weeks

SCENARIO OVERVIEW: Chlorine gas is poisonous and can be pressurized and cooled to change it into a liquid form so that it can be shipped and stored. When released, it quickly turns into a gas and stays close to the ground and spreads rapidly. Chlorine gas is yellow-green in color and although not flammable alone, it can react explosively or form explosive compounds with other chemicals such as turpentine or ammonia. In this scenario, the Universal Adversary (UA) infiltrates an industrial facility and stores a large quantity of chlorine gas (liquefied under pressure). Using a low-order explosive, UA ruptures a storage tank man-way, releasing a large quantity of chlorine gas downwind of the site. Secondary devices are set to impact first responders.

Natural Disaster 9

Major Earthquake

CASUALTIES: 1,400 fatalities; 100,000 hospitalizations
INFRASTRUCTURE DAMAGE: 150,000 buildings destroyed, 1 million buildings damaged
EVACUATIONS/DISPLACED PERSONS: 300,000 households
CONTAMINATION: from hazardous materials, in some areas
ECONOMIC IMPACT: hundreds of billions
POTENTIAL FOR MULTIPLE EVENTS: yes, aftershocks
RECOVERY TIMELINE: months to years

SCENARIO OVERVIEW: When plates that form under the Earth's surface suddenly shift an earthquake can occur. The magnitude of an earthquake is measured by the amplitude of the seismic waves. A quake of magnitude 2 is the smallest quake normally felt by people. Earthquakes measuring 6 or higher are commonly considered major. In this scenario, a 7.2-magnitude earthquake occurs along a fault zone in a major metropolitan area (MMA) of a city, greatly impacting a six-county region with a population of approximately 10 million people. Subsurface faulting occurs along 45 miles of the fault zone, extending along a large portion of highly populated local jurisdictions, creating a large swath of destruction. Soil liquefaction occurs and creates quicksand-like conditions.

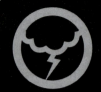

Natural Disaster 10

Major Hurricane

CASUALTIES: 1,000 fatalities, 5,000 hospitalizations
INFRASTRUCTURE DAMAGE: buildings destroyed, large debris
EVACUATIONS/DISPLACED PERSONS: 1 million evacuated; 100,000 homes seriously damaged
CONTAMINATION: From hazardous materials, in some areas
ECONOMIC IMPACT: millions of dollars
POTENTIAL FOR MULTIPLE EVENTS: yes, seasonal
RECOVERY TIMELINE: months

SCENARIO OVERVIEW: Hurricanes are tropical weather systems producing dangerous winds, torrential rains, and storm surges up to 24 feet high and 100 miles wide. Hurricane force winds cover 400 miles in diameter. "Major" hurricanes are placed in Categories 3, 4, or 5 with sustained wind intensities in excess of 155 mph. The most dangerous storm is a slow-moving Category 5 hurricane, making landfall in a highly populated area. In this scenario, a Category 5 hurricane hits a major metropolitan area (MMA). Sustained winds are at 160 mph with a storm surge greater than 20 feet above normal. As the storm moves closer, massive evacuations are required. Some escape routes are flooded five hours before the eye of the hurricane reaches land.

Radiological Attack 11

Radiological Dispersal Devices

CASUALTIES: 180 fatalities; 270 injuries; 20,000 detectible contaminations (at each site)
INFRASTRUCTURE DAMAGE: near the explosion
EVACUATIONS/DISPLACED PERSONS: yes
CONTAMINATION: 36 city blocks (at each site)
ECONOMIC IMPACT: up to billions of dollars
POTENTIAL FOR MULTIPLE EVENTS: yes
RECOVERY TIMELINE: months to years

SCENARIO OVERVIEW: Cesium-137 (137Cs) decays by beta and gamma radiation and stands out as a radioactive isotope highly suitable for radiological terror. This isotope causes skin damage similar to burns and would be particularly dangerous if accidentally ingested or inhaled. In this scenario, the Universal Adversary (UA) detonates "dirty bombs" of 137Cs in three regionally close, moderate-to-large cities. The contaminated region covers approximately thirty-six blocks in each city. The entire scene is contaminated with 137Cs. The size of most of the particles is approximately 100 microns. Larger particles either penetrate building materials in the blast zone or drop to the ground as fall-out. Wind patterns carry the contamination in unpredictable directions and air intakes contaminate interiors of larger buildings and subway systems.

Explosives Attack 12

Improvised Bombs

CASUALTIES: 100 fatalities; 450 hospitalizations
INFRASTRUCTURE DAMAGE: structures affected by blast and fire
EVACUATIONS/DISPLACED PERSONS: minimal
CONTAMINATION: none
ECONOMIC IMPACT: local
POTENTIAL FOR MULTIPLE EVENTS: yes
RECOVERY TIMELINE: weeks to months

SCENARIO OVERVIEW: In this scenario, agents of the Universal Adversary (UA) use improvised explosive devices (IEDs) to detonate bombs inside a sports arena and create a large vehicle bomb (LVB). They also use suicide bombers in an underground public transportation concourse and detonate another bomb in a parking facility near the entertainment complex. An additional series of devices is detonated in the lobby of the nearest hospital emergency room (ER). The event is primarily designed for an urban environment, but could be adapted for more rural area events such as county fairs and other large gatherings. Casualty estimates would be reduced as a function of a reduced target population and less population density at target points.

CHAPTER 5 — MANAGE RISK

Biological Attack 13

Food Contamination

CASUALTIES: 300 fatalities; 400 hospitalizations
INFRASTRUCTURE DAMAGE: none
EVACUATIONS/DISPLACED PERSONS: none
CONTAMINATION: sites where contamination was dispersed
ECONOMIC IMPACT: millions of dollars
POTENTIAL FOR MULTIPLE EVENTS: yes
RECOVERY TIMELINE: weeks

SCENARIO OVERVIEW: The U.S. food industry has significantly increased its physical and personnel security since 2001. However, in this scenario the Universal Adversary (UA) is able to acquire restricted documents due to a security lapse. The UA uses these sensitive documents to conduct a serious attack. The UA delivers liquid anthrax bacteria to pre-selected plant workers. At a beef plant in a west coast state, two batches of ground beef are contaminated with anthrax with distribution to a west coast city, a southwest state, and a state in the northwest. At an orange juice plant in a southwestern state, three batches of orange juice are contaminated with anthrax, with distribution to a west coast city, a southwest city, and a northwest city.

Biological Attack 14

Foreign Animal Disease (Foot & Mouth disease)

CASUALTIES: none
INFRASTRUCTURE DAMAGE: huge loss of livestock
EVACUATIONS/DISPLACED PERSONS: up to 70,000 (self evacuate)
CONTAMINATION: none
ECONOMIC IMPACT: hundreds of millions of dollars
POTENTIAL FOR MULTIPLE EVENTS: yes
RECOVERY TIMELINE: months

SCENARIO OVERVIEW: Foot and mouth disease is an acute infectious viral disease that causes blisters, fever, and lameness in cloven-hoofed animals such as cattle and swine. The disease is not considered a human threat. In this scenario, members of the Universal Adversary (UA) enter the United States to survey large operations in the livestock industries. The UA targets several locations for a coordinated bioterrorism attack on the agricultural industry. Approximately two months later, UA teams enter the United States and infect farm animals at specific locations. Although the initial event will be localized at transportation facilities in several states, as the biological agent matures and the livestock are transported, the geographical area will widen to include surrounding states where the livestock are delivered.

Cyber Attack 15

Cyber Attack

CASUALTIES: none directly
INFRASTRUCTURE DAMAGE: cyber
EVACUATIONS/DISPLACED PERSONS: none
CONTAMINATION: none
ECONOMIC IMPACT: millions of dollars
POTENTIAL FOR MULTIPLE EVENTS: yes
RECOVERY TIMELINE: weeks

SCENARIO OVERVIEW: In this scenario, the Universal Adversary conducts cyber attacks that affect several parts of the nation's financial infrastructure over the course of several weeks. Specifically, credit-card processing facilities are hacked and numbers are released to the Internet, causing 20 million cards to be cancelled; automated teller machines (ATMs) fail across the nation; major companies report payroll checks were not received; several large pension and mutual fund companies have computer malfunctions so severe that they are unable to operate for more than a week. Individually, these attacks are not dangerous, but combined, they shatter faith in the stability of the system. Citizens no longer trust any part of the U.S. financial system and foreign speculators make a run on the dollar.

CHAPTER 5 — MANAGE RISK

A COLLABORATIVE CHOICE

Regardless of the method used to organize information about threats and vulnerabilities, choosing which risks to prioritize requires collaboration with other preparedness professions.

No *single* preparedness profession is likely to prevent catastrophe on its own. Response and recovery do not fall to a single profession. A collaborative choice is the only practical choice.

Unless local preparedness professions share authentic ownership of the risk priorities, they are unlikely to direct their independent resources toward prevention, response, and recovery in accordance with the priorities.

The risk priorities do not have to be a consensus choice. Elected leaders or their delegates may make the final decision. But the preparedness professions must understand how the priorities were selected and have confidence in the process of selection. Otherwise the significant independence—and turf consciousness—of the preparedness professions will undermine meaningful attention to any priority.

Wide distribution of the same intelligence products among the preparedness professions is one way of producing a collaborative choice. Welcoming contributions from all of the preparedness professions in developing the intelligence products also helps. Bringing the preparedness professions together to identify threats is an important first step for any kind of collaboration.

Complementing "expert panel" assessments of vulnerability, threat, and consequences with "practitioner panels"—with members from all the preparedness professions—is another productive method of producing a collaborative choice.

Working through the DHS planning scenarios is an excellent way of building collaborative connections and beginning to share the key elements of a collaborative choice.

In making a collaborative choice, it is important that the community not settle for a

No single preparedness profession is likely to prevent catastrophe on its own.

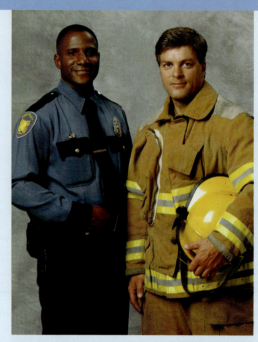

Source: PhotoDisc

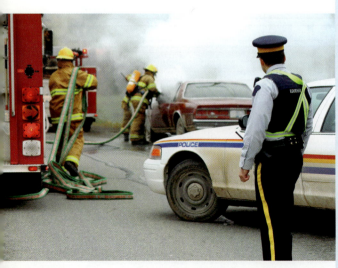

Source: iStockphoto

compromise choice. The goal is to identify the catastrophic risk or risks facing your community. **The goal has nothing to do with selecting those risks that best justify existing budget requests.** Your community's most serious risks may compete with existing priorities. There will be a tendency for the collaborative process to make choices that reinforce continued collaboration. But collaboration is not the goal. Collaboration is a means to achieving the goal of effectively managing risk.

Collaborative decision-making can benefit from involvement of a "**devil's advocate**" or a "**china-breaker**." This is usually someone from outside the collaborative process who is involved specifically to keep decision-makers away from self-justifying choices. A paid consultant, a retired preparedness professional from another community or similar outsider is important to involve so that tough collaboration does not descend into easy compromise.

In most communities, the choice of the top risk priority or even top three risk priorities is a judgment call. It is a tough call. The choice is only worthwhile to the extent the preparedness professions support the choice. Involving the preparedness professions in choosing the risk priority is time-consuming and sometimes contentious, but it is also just about the only way to produce decisions that gain traction.

*In making a collaborative choice, it is important that the community not make what is just a **compromise** choice.*

If you had just enough budget to invite **ten local people** to a start-up meeting for a collaborative process in risk management, whom would you invite?

1 _____
2 _____
3 _____
4 _____
5 _____
6 _____
7 _____
8 _____
9 _____
10 _____

Do you know someone who would be good at the role of a "china-breaker" during collaborative decision making? (circle one)

yes   no

If yes, who? _____

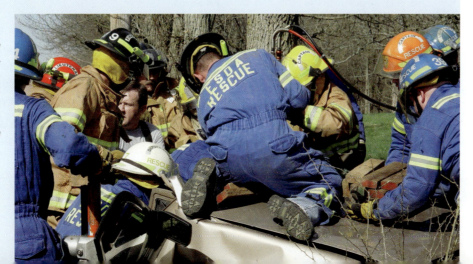

*Sangamon County Rescue Squad, New Berlin Fire Department, and other Central Illinois emergency response agencies work collaboratively in response to a vehicle crash.
Source: Photo by Jerry McKay, Sangamon County Rescue Squad*

TARA: FOUR RESPONSES TO RISK

Once you have identified your risk priorities there is a need to decide how to manage them. The insurance and risk management industries have found there are **four choices available regarding any risk:**

TRANSFER: Is there a way to transfer the risk from one place to another? For natural threats, building dams and levees to control flooding in one part of a river can increase the risks of flooding downstream. For intentional threats, because terrorists are strategic actors they will often prefer less protected targets. By choosing to increase protection at one target, you are probably transferring risk to another target. You may, for example, choose to increase protection at a chemical plant in an effort to transfer the risk to what you believe will be a target with less catastrophic potential.

AVOID: Is there a way to simply avoid the risk? An example is to use zoning laws to restrict construction in a flood plain. In this way the risk of future flooding is avoided. In some cases avoidance of risk also involves reducing or eliminating opportunities. As a result, not all risks are considered prudent to avoid.

REDUCE: Is there a way to mitigate the severity of potential loss? You might build redundant systems. You might increase investment in response capabilities. You might disperse your critical infrastructure. You might decentralize key services and processes. How can you reduce the threat by reducing your vulnerabilities?

ACCEPT: Many times we choose to accept the risk. In terms of risk management, it is very important that this is a conscious choice, explicitly made, and as a result ready for explicit review and, if appropriate, revision.

Your community will accept several risks. Many of these risks you would prefer not to accept. Unfortunately, given resources available and your assessment of other risks, risk acceptance is often a reasonable choice.

Each risk—each unique combination of threat, vulnerability, and consequence—can be managed differently. Application of TARA to an earthquake is very different than application to a terrorist threat. Application of TARA to many threat capabilities, on the other hand, may be similar. Whether a wild fire is started by lightning, an errant cigarette, or a terrorist is unlikely to change your risk analysis or your risk management choices. Application of TARA to a short-term situation—such as a major sporting or political event—is likely to be very different than application to a long-term vulnerability such as being located on the coast in hurricane country. Application of TARA to a place with a highly concentrated population is usually different than application to a sparsely populated place.

A collaborative process for choosing to transfer, avoid, reduce or accept your major risk priorities will, once again, reinforce the likelihood that these choices actually influence the strategic and operational decisions of all of the preparedness professions.

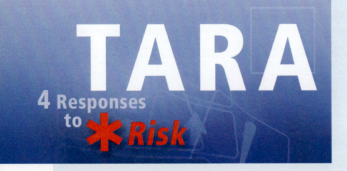

TARA

4 Responses to *Risk

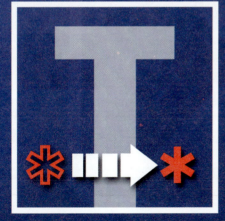
TRANSFER

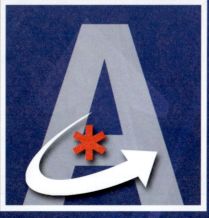
AVOID

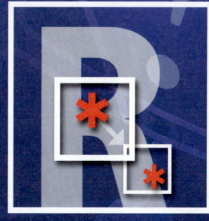
REDUCE

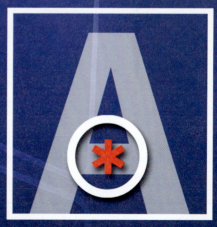
ACCEPT

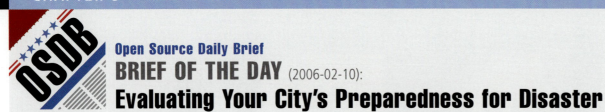

Open Source Daily Brief
BRIEF OF THE DAY (2006-02-10):
Evaluating Your City's Preparedness for Disaster

The American Disaster Preparedness Foundation recently completed a study of the preparedness of the largest metropolitan areas in the United States. The mission of the American Disaster Preparedness Foundation (ADPF), an Illinois non-profit public advocacy organization, is to help ensure that the American public prepares adequately for disasters.

The study measured nine specific factors, including:
(1) Technology,
(2) Management,
(3) Maintenance,
(4) Infrastructure,
(5) Internal Training,
(6) Equity,
(7) Public Education,
(8) General Awareness, and
(9) External Support.

Each city received a letter grade corresponding to the numerical score from the evaluation.

In general, the scores from the study indicate a poor level of preparedness for disaster response efforts in the future, unless significant improvements occur in emergency planning. The highest-ranking city, Phoenix, received only a B+ and more than half of all major metropolitan cities in the study rated worse than a C.

Four primary findings of the study revealed:

- The Midwest is the least prepared region of the United States
- The West Coast and Florida are the most prepared regions
- No single major metropolitan area satisfactorily addresses the needs of the disabled, elderly, or the poor
- Even the best public disaster education programs evaluated are weak; some programs are almost non-existent

An efficient response to a disaster requires cooperation between government officials and first responders. Ordinary residents, however, also play an important role. The knowledge and skill of residents in handling themselves and their families during an emergency affects the overall level of preparedness of each metro area. For example, if an area's evacuation plan has the chief goal of requiring residents to "shelter in place," citizens must know how to do so effectively.

Preparedness and prevention go hand-in-hand. The ADPF research supports the conclusion that the nation's ability to mitigate disasters effectively requires a higher level of preparedness of individuals, communities, cities, states, and the federal government. The study done by ADPF provides a comparative assessment of preparedness, and a baseline to use in measuring future advances.

PREVENTION RELEVANCE: Preparedness and prevention go hand-in-hand. The former mitigates the harm caused when the latter fails.

PREVENTION TECHNIQUES: Measure your city's current level of preparedness to establish a baseline. Define the areas that need restructuring or additional development. Write and implement a performance improvement plan. Evaluate the improvements and measure them against the original baseline.

PREVENTION THOUGHT: Risk Management
Does your city have an emergency management plan? Are all the key players identified and properly trained?

The Open Source Daily Brief is a service of the Institute for Preventive Strategies (©IPS). You can register to receive the OSDBs at www.preventivestrategies.net.

CONTINUALLY ASSESS YOUR CHOICE

Stuff happens. Things change. It is important to continue monitoring your situation for new threats, new vulnerabilities, and changes in old threats and vulnerabilities. It is important to have a process in place to adjust which risks you consider a priority and how you plan to manage the risks.

Your community's strategic intelligence function is crucial to this ability to assess—and potentially change—your perceptions of risk and decisions about how to manage risk.

Precisely how you do this largely depends on how your community currently chooses and manages other priorities. It will also depend on how successful you are in developing an effective collaborative process to choose your risk priorities and manage these risks.

But **at a minimum, your strategic intelligence function needs to review the risk management priorities on a monthly basis.** An explicit judgment is necessary on whether the current priorities match the threat environment and current vulnerabilities.

If the strategic intelligence function suggests adjusting risk management priorities, there should be a procedure by which the collaborative partners can respond quickly to changing circumstance. The risk formula is helpful in this assessment.

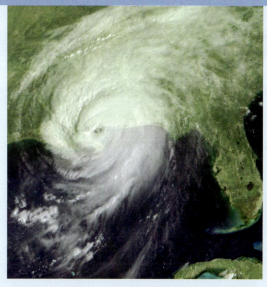

ABOVE: *Hurricane Katrina, 2005; satellite imagery. Source: NASA's Earth Observatory, nasa.gov*

Consequence is closely related to Likelihood (threat and vulnerability). Consequences often change depending on the specific time and place of the threat. Vulnerability can be especially influenced by time and place. For example, the threat of a hurricane is seasonal. What may be a significant Likelihood in July is much lower in December. The vulnerability associated with a major music festival bringing thousands of participants to a particular location for a few days quickly reduces when the music festival ends.

Tracking changes in threat and vulnerability helps in regularly assessing shifts that could challenge the basic assumptions used in your risk management priorities.

Given your current perception of your community's catastrophic risk, which risk management choice has been made?

Has this been a conscious choice or a choice emerging from neglect?

Do you personally support this choice?

CHAPTER 5 — MANAGE RISK

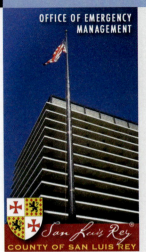

San Luis Rey® is a fictional jurisdiction designed by Teleologic Learning LLC. All characters, locations, and events are fictitious and intended for instructional purposes only.

COUNTY OF SAN LUIS REY®
OFFICE OF EMERGENCY MANAGEMENT

RESULTS OF THE ALL-HAZARDS RISK ASSESSMENT

A county risk assessment has been completed in cooperation with the State of Hamilton, the Cities of San Luis Rey, Juniper Shore, Lakeview, Northfield, and Port Estaban, the San Luis Rey Port Authority, Lake Juniper Water Authority, San Luis Rey State University, the Federal Bureau of Investigation, and the Regional Commission on Economic Development. The following is only a summary.

The Office of Emergency Management expresses its appreciation to the cooperating parties and all of those who participated in the Delphi Analysis.

Decision-makers should be aware that Likelihood is a factor that can change quickly. This factor is determined by an assessment of threat and vulnerability. As such, new information can have a significant impact on the analysis. Accordingly, the Office of Emergency Management will continue to work with the cooperating agencies to regularly assess and update the risk assessment.

Further related to Likelihood, the risk management process has encouraged the OEM to regularly update all cooperating agencies on the current mode of the identified risk: primary, secondary, or tertiary. The shift of a risk from primary mode into secondary or tertiary should be used by the cooperating agencies to adjust deployment of assets accordingly.

Priority Risks	Capability-Based Summary (initial Impacts)	Likelihood (Delphi Average of 1-10)	Potential Consequences (Delphi Average of 1-10)	Risk Factor (LxC=Risk)
1. Hurricane	death, flooding, severe structural damage, major infrastructure compromised	8.9	7.2	86.08
2. Toxic Chemical Release	death, blindness, neurological trauma, long-term ecological contamination	9.1	5.0	53.60
3. Radiological/Nuclear Event	death, genetic damage severe structural damage, long-term human contamination	5.1	8.9	45.39
4. Pandemic	death and debilitation	6.2	7.6	47.12
5. Terrorist Attack	varied kinetic impacts potentially replicating any of the foregoing	6.1	5.3	32.33

How would the risk priorities change if credible intelligence indicated a terrorist capability to weaponize smallpox?

If a terrorist attack, successful or not, was launched on a nuclear power station in Britain, how would this (should this) impact the list of risk priorities above? (San Luis Rey has a nuclear power station.)

If the intentional threat of terrorism "replicates" (repeats, copies, is the same as) the other priority risks, how should this influence the priority your community gives to counter-terrorism and anti-terrorism work?

MANAGE RISK:
Chapter Review

Do the current priorities of your fire service agency complement or compete with risk management of catastrophe? How so?

_____
_____
_____
_____
_____
_____
_____

What two elements interact to produce Likelihood in the risk formula:

Likelihood x Consequences = Risk

_____
_____
_____
_____
_____

How do the two elements that determine Likelihood interact?

_____
_____
_____
_____
_____
_____

In the risk formula, Likelihood x Consequences = Risk, consequences will almost always determine which likelihood is chosen as the highest risk. Why? Do you agree that this is appropriate?

_____
_____
_____
_____
_____
_____
_____
_____
_____
_____

Which of the 15 DHS planning scenarios do you consider most relevant to your community?

_____
_____
_____
_____
_____
_____
_____

What technique can be used to help ensure that collaboration continues to focus on risk management rather than political compromise?

_____
_____
_____
_____
_____

What does each letter in the TARA acronym stand for?

T _____

A _____

R _____

A _____

How often should your community's risk management priorities be reviewed?

_____
_____
_____
_____

What risk factors should be monitored for change to determine the need to adjust your community's risk priorities?

_____
_____
_____
_____
_____
_____
_____

CHAPTER 5 — MANAGE RISK

APPLY WHAT YOU HAVE LEARNED

Use your CD to access the Risk Management Advanced Exercise. Select the **Chapter 5** Certificate Course link located in the Online Exercises section of your CD.

By now you have gained a familiarity with the principles of developing threat and vulnerability assessments. You have recognized the need to collaborate in order to gather, analyze and share information. In this chapter of the workbook you have been exposed to some algorithms for deciding what the acceptable risks are.

In this exercise you will find that the San Luis Rey terrorists are continuing to plan and execute. **It is now about 3 months before the attack.**

You too have been busy. As a Senior Captain in the San Luis Rey Fire Department, you have spearheaded threat and vulnerability assessments, developed an effective collaboration network, and established strategic information sharing channels that provide you the strategic intelligence you will need to determine the risks associated with this threat.

Your hard work has paid off. **Now you and your team are ready to identify and assess the risks associated with this threat.** You will continue to utilize your collaboration and information sharing networks to establish your risk management strategy, and to hone your sense of the threat and prioritize the risks.

Note: If you have already enrolled in the Homeland Security Terrorism Prevention Certificate Course for Fire Service Professionals (©IPS) you can go directly to the exercise by using the Online Exercises Direct Access links on your CD or by typing this URL into your browser's address window:

www.preventivestrategies.net/go/ mhfs-adv-ex-manage-risk

For first time access, use this initial URL:
www.preventivestrategies.net/go/ mhfs-enroll

Three San Luis Rey Senior Fire Captains will present their risk management strategies. Can you correctly identify their strengths and weaknesses?

The clock is still ticking…

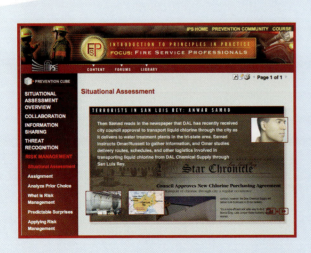
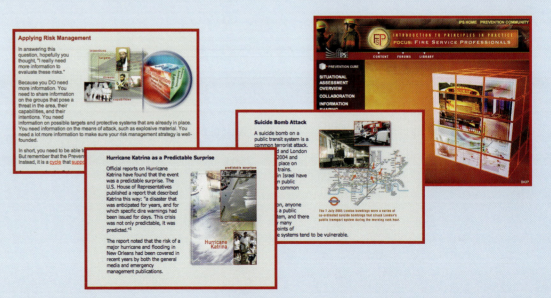

San Luis Rey® is a fictional jurisdiction designed by Teleologic Learning LLC. All characters, locations, and events are fictitious and intended for instructional purposes only.

Decide to Intervene

✓ *In this chapter you will learn:*
- How to apply the principles of protection, deterrence, and preemption.
- How to determine if you are dealing with a risk in its primary, secondary, or tertiary mode.
- How to make an effective decision.
- How to utilize the outcomes of effective risk management to support your community's application for federal funding.

In tactical operations, there can sometimes be little difference between scanning, analyzing, and responding. The more urgent the response the more likely the first three steps are compressed into one step.

With a strategic goal it is possible—and helpful—to be very clear about each step and to add assessment. Prevention of catastrophe is a strategic goal. **The basics of SARA apply to this goal.**

In **collaboration** with others, you **scan** the strategic horizon and **share information** on threats and vulnerabilities.

In collaboration with others, you **analyze** the information you have shared and **identify** both **specific threats** and **threat capabilities.**

In collaboration with others, you **respond** by deciding to **manage risk** by choosing which risks will receive priority attention.

In collaboration with others, you assess and **decide whether to intervene and how**: you choose how to respond to the risks.

What will you and your collaborative partners do?

In what sequence will you do it?

Talk it through, plan it, train it, exercise it, do it, and **assess** it.

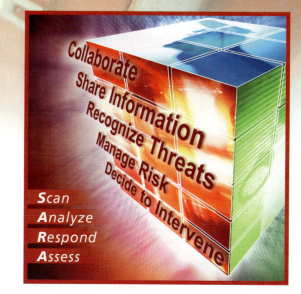

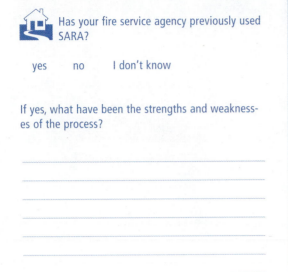

Has your fire service agency previously used SARA?

yes   no   I don't know

If yes, what have been the strengths and weaknesses of the process?

_____
_____
_____
_____
_____
_____

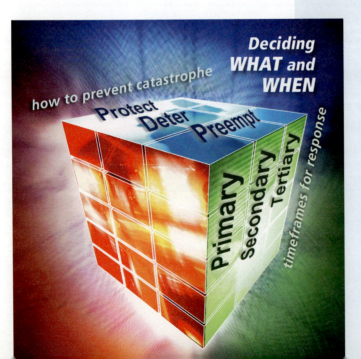

THE PREVENTION CUBE: WHAT AND WHEN?

The prevention cube provides a framework for fire service professionals to use in thinking about the problem of catastrophic risk, whether natural, accidental, or intentional. It exemplifies the relationships between analytic processes, types of intervention, and modes of intervention in prevention activities.

The **top face** of the prevention cube suggests the **types of intervention** involved in preparing for, and preventing, catastrophe:

To **Protect** is to make people and places less vulnerable through vaccinations, shielding, environmental and architectural design, surveillance, and other technological means.

To **Deter** is to influence the thinking of those who threaten the community. For example, deterrence in one area may shift terrorist attention to "softer" targets. This is called "displacement."

To **Preempt** is to take action during the earliest stages of a threatening event to detect and stop it.

Protection is possible for natural, accidental, and intentional threats. Deterrence is usually not associated with natural threats, but is useful against both accidental and intentional threats. Preemption is especially effective with intentional threats. Preemption is less likely with most natural and accidental threats.

The **side** of **the prevention cube** shows **three timeframes, or modes, for intervening.** These can also be thought of as phases. Each timeframe represents a different level of urgency. It is possible to preempt, deter, and protect in each timeframe. The type of preemption, deterrence, and protection will differ depending on the urgency of the risk.

- **Primary mode intervention:** Intervening to reduce risk before knowing about a specific threat, but after a threat capability is recognized. Primary mode intervention activities correspond roughly to those preparedness and prevention measures involved in general operations. For example, a community engages in hurricane risk reduction before the beginning of hurricane season.

- **Secondary mode intervention:** Intervening after a potential specific threat is recognized but before there is evidence of an immediate threat. Secondary mode intervention activities correspond roughly to operational measures involved in preparing for, and preventing, specifically recognized threats. For example, a tropical storm is forming in the mid-Atlantic.

- **Tertiary mode intervention:** Intervening because a recognized threat poses a clear-and-present danger. Tertiary mode intervention activities correspond roughly to those preparedness and prevention measures involved in either mitigating or preempting a recognized threat. For example, participation in evacuation of an area could result from the National Hurricane Center identifying your community as being in the path of a specific hurricane's landfall zone.

The same time sensitive—or phase sensitive—approach is useful in preparing for, and preventing, natural, accidental, and intentional threats. It is the threat capability of a hurricane for which a community prepares. Whether it is Hurricane Agnes or Greg does not really matter. The same capability-based planning is useful against every kind of threat.

Deciding what you will do when—and ensuring that the decisions are actually carried out—**begins to translate your risk management choices into actionable decisions.**

PRIMARY MODE: PROTECT, DETER, AND PREEMPT

If you have invested in collaborating to share information, recognize threats, and manage risks you should be able to make good decisions about how to prevent catastrophe.

As the scenario-based assessment process demonstrates, many natural, accidental, and intentional threats share a similar threat capability. **By reducing your community's vulnerability to any of these capabilities you reduce vulnerability to all of the threats. By reducing your own vulnerability to threats, you ensure your department's capability to manage the full range of natural, accidental, and intentional threats.**

For example, many experts think the catastrophic impact of Hurricane Katrina on New Orleans was preventable. Several studies suggested that building and maintaining the existing protections well would have reduced the flooding. Several studies suggest preservation of delta marshland could have substantially reduced the hurricane's impact. If these studies are accurate, it is an especially good example of the importance of giving priority to long-term prevention and risk management.

Reducing vulnerability is often achieved through protection. An increased police presence may protect the target of an intentional threat. For example, in at least one case a terrorist plan to attack New York City bridges was discouraged by an increased level of police protection. Increased "hardening" can also protect physical structures. Building codes in many hurricane and earthquake prone areas are much more rigorous—and vigorously enforced—than in other areas. In the case of accidental threats, protection might include buffer zones between chemical plants, refineries, or similar facilities and residential areas, schools, hospitals, and other "targets" of an accidental catastrophe.

Zoning, building codes, and other policy oriented protective measures often take years—even decades—to become fully effective. Yet, owners and managers of facilities that store, handle, and transport Hazmat often welcome local fire department efforts to collaborate and share information about operational safety and security. The fact that the federal government considers the petrochemical industry part of the critical infrastructure of the United States makes it increasingly important for fire departments to gather information about local vulnerabilities related to the industry. How familiar is your department with the industrial sites in your response district that store, handle, or transport Hazmat?

The Local Emergency Planning Commission (LEPC) provision of the Clean Air Act provides an LEPC database along with a

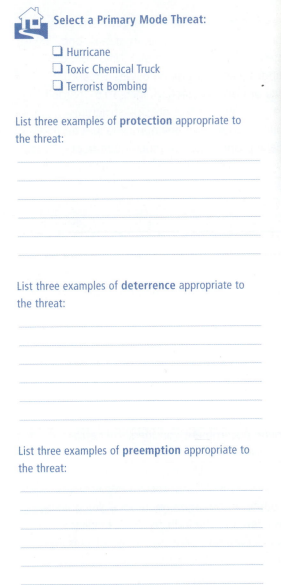

Select a Primary Mode Threat:

❑ Hurricane
❑ Toxic Chemical Truck
❑ Terrorist Bombing

List three examples of **protection** appropriate to the threat:

_____
_____
_____
_____
_____
_____

List three examples of **deterrence** appropriate to the threat:

_____
_____
_____
_____
_____
_____

List three examples of **preemption** appropriate to the threat:

_____
_____
_____
_____
_____
_____

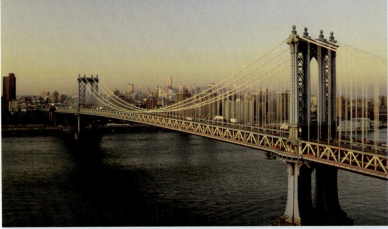

A terrorist plan to attack New York City bridges was discouraged by an increased level of police protection.

Manhattan Bridge, New York City.
Source: ablestock.com

search capability to display information about 3000 listings across the United States. See the CD for a link to the LEPC database. In addition, your fire marshal or inspector can arrange to visit facilities for a range of purposes, to do an inspection or to collaborate. Sources of information that may prove helpful include the **material safety data sheets (MSDS)** for the Hazmat stored, handled, or transported at the facility. **Each MSDS outlines the following types of information:**

- **The chemical's known health hazards**
- **Properties of the material (both physical and chemical)**
- **First aid procedures**
- **Firefighting recommendations**
- **Protective clothing/equipment requirements**
- **Emergency telephone contact numbers**

Taking protective action in collaboration with local facilities that store, handle, or transport Hazmat also involves sharing information about risk management techniques used. The on-site coordinator or safety manager can often provide Process Safety Management (PSM) scenario information on potential consequences expected from an accidental release.

However, Craig Shelley and Anthony Cole point out, "release and consequence scenarios for accidental releases may not be as severe as those for a terrorist-related release" (p. 64). The existing safety regulations for facilities that store, handle, or transport Hazmat do not cover security issues related to preventing intentional threats. Congress recently addressed this deficiency by providing the Department of Homeland Security (DHS) with the authority to regulate certain high-risk chemical facilities.

Section 550 of the Homeland Security Appropriations Act of 2007 ("Section 550") provides DHS with authority to develop "interim final regulations" regarding security of certain chemical facilities in the United States. (See link on the CD.) Though it is unclear what security standards DHS will require from high-risk chemical facilities, this new area of regulation poses additional opportunities for the fire service to engage the business community to better understand vulnerabilities and potential protective measures.

Fire service organizations must also protect their own capabilities if they are to remain prepared to respond effectively to catastrophic events. Among all the preparatory efforts, the most basic one of all is to **maintain preplans for family members in case of a catastrophe**. Fire service agencies protect themselves through a range of operational security measures and response preparedness planning and training.

Primary mode measures focused on preserving fire service capabilities include:
- Safeguarding assets such as apparatus and equipment
- Maintaining access control to facilities
- Assigning personnel to observe visitors and manage their movement through facilities
- Maintaining a visitor log recording names, addresses, and phone numbers
- Reporting any documents present at an incident that include diagrams, drawings, or photographs of potential or identified targets, especially when written in a foreign language
- Refining and exercising preplans involving multiagency response
- Maintaining preplans for family members in case of a catastrophe
- Maintaining a Critical Incident Stress Management Plan (CISM) for the department
- Maintaining a Continuity of Operations (COOP) Plan
- Institutionalizing ongoing vulnerability assessments
- Maintaining ongoing communications checks with emergency response and command locations
- Maintaining mutual aid agreements, keeping all critical information current
- Regularly monitoring intelligence reports from local and national sources, both classified and open source
- Reporting any suspicious situations to the appropriate authorities

(See *Fire and Emergency Services Preparedness Guide…*)

Deterrence is typically a police function. The increased protection of New York City bridges, noted above, served to deter. The police protection persuaded terrorists to look for easier targets. Education and training can also deter accidents. Anything that influences the thinking behind a potential threat is a form of deterrence. Some have speculated that aggressive enforcement of fire and building codes could have a deterrent effect.

Others argue terrorism is not deterred but displaced. Terrorists may simply look for another target. In some special cases, deterrence may actually attract attention. The first

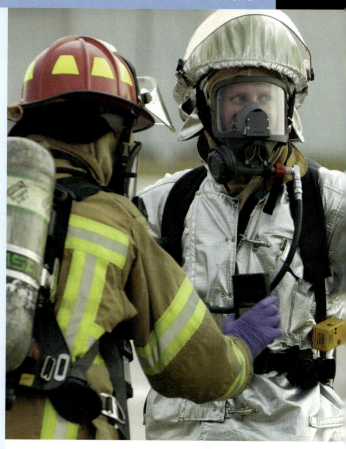

A firefighter with Jacksonville Fire and Rescue Department checks U.S. Air Force Staff Sgt. Stephen Ingrando, a firefighter with 125th Fighter Wing, Florida National Guard, for exposure to chemical and radiological agents during the tri-annual mass casualty exercise at the Jacksonville International Airport, Florida; 2006.
Source: DoDMedia photo by Staff Sgt Shelley Gill

Take protective action in collaboration with local facilities that store, handle, or transport Hazmat.

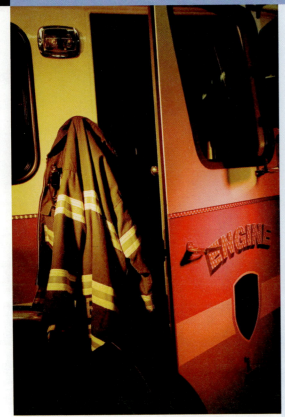

Source: iStockphoto

Fire service organizations must protect their own assets and capabilities if they are to remain prepared to respond effectively to catastrophic events.

terrorist attack on the World Trade Center in 1993 was only partially successful. The trial of those involved in the first attack was almost complete in the late summer of 2001. The decision to attack the WTC towers was, in part, a public declaration of being undeterred.

Because earthquakes, hurricanes, and other natural threats are unthinking, we generally do not consider deterrence as preventing or mitigating these threats. Nevertheless, education, training, and other preparation can increase the public's resilience regarding natural threats. In this way, we work to "deter" the outcomes of natural threats even if we cannot deter the threat itself. Having emergency supplies on hand, being aware of evacuation measures, and knowing where and how to get accurate information can all work to prevent or reduce the consequences of natural, accidental, or intentional threats.

The fire department—or even the well timed use of a garden hose—can preempt a wild fire in its earliest stages. We cannot preempt hurricanes, tornadoes, earthquakes, floods and most other sources of natural catastrophe. Once they start, these threats play out regardless of what we do.

We can sometimes preempt an accidental threat. A quick response very early in an accident can serve to reverse the threat or—at least—tightly contain it. The success of preemption is often directly tied to training operators and first responders, and their ability to accurately recognize and quickly respond to an accident. On the other hand, active engagement with owners and managers of facilities storing, handling, or transporting Hazmat can augment the "safety culture" in those enterprises and lower the likelihood of decisions to cut corners on safety and security.

We can preempt an intentional threat early in its planning stages. Often this is the result of intelligence operations exposing a specific threat. We can disrupt a terrorist operation with sufficiently specific tactical intelligence before an attack. An effective fire investigation can apprehend a serial arsonist.

Yet, even without specific intelligence, vigilant law enforcement or citizen involvement can recognize early signs and signals and take preemptive action. Noticing a suspicious driver at a Washington State ferry crossing preempted a New Year's 2000 attack.

The fire service can play a critically important role in primary mode prevention by actively taking part in developing and enforcing performance-based building codes. These standards can—if thoughtfully adopted and applied—enhance the entire community's understanding of risk and the role of community-wide decision-making related to risk. But performance-based building codes—as with most risk-based decision-making—require ongoing review and revision. Adopting some version of a performance-based code is not a one-time fix. Firefighters have the expertise and credibility to help the public and elected officials understand the benefits and the limitations of performance-based building codes.

In the United States there are two competing Model Codes that each use performance-based standards. Information on the International Building Code (IBC) is available from the International Code Council (http://www.iccsafe.org/). Information on the Comprehensive Consensus Codes (C3) is available from the National Fire Protection Association (http://www.nfpa.org).

A sometimes-critical analysis of performance-based building codes is available from the National Institutes of Standards and Technology. This publication, *Evolution of Performance Based Codes and Fire Safety Design Methods*, is available on your CD.

During routine operations, firefighters can remain aware of a range of suspicious situations they may see, such as:

- Presence in an occupancy of hardcopy, or electronic, materials profiling important U.S. officials, facilities, security points, etc.
- Presence in an occupancy of detailed diagrams and notes about buildings, ports, bridges
- Out of place chemicals in an occupancy
- Multiple copies of passports, driver's licenses, or other official documents with the same person's picture
- Asking any visitors who want detailed information why they are interested, especially if they are taking detailed notes using audio or video recordings:
  - gauging their response (such information might include requests for the gross vehicle weight of an apparatus, or how many people can ride in it)
  - requesting that anyone who seems offended take a photograph with you, making sure to use the department's camera
  - sharing all the information collected about suspicious visitors to the appropriate law enforcement agency

(Welch; and Martinez and McLoughlin)

SECONDARY MODE:
PROTECT, DETER, AND PREEMPT

In the primary mode, you feel great but know that heart disease runs in your family. In the secondary mode, you feel great but are overweight and your bad cholesterol is higher than recommended. In the secondary mode, there is a much greater vulnerability. The risk of harm is significantly elevated.

In the primary mode hurricane season is six months away. In the secondary mode, a tropical depression is forming in the Atlantic. In the primary mode, terrorism is a national

> What are examples of **deterrence** that your fire service agency has used in dealing with non-catastrophic threats?

Select a Secondary Mode Threat:

❏ Earthquake
❏ Accidental Release of Toxin
❏ Terrorist Cyberattack

List three examples of **protection** appropriate to the threat:

_____
_____
_____
_____

List three examples of **deterrence** appropriate to the threat:

_____
_____
_____
_____

List three examples of **preemption** appropriate to the threat:

_____
_____
_____
_____

concern and there is a terrorist capability that puts your community at risk. In the secondary mode, you have strategic intelligence that suggests terrorists have recently enhanced their biological attack capability using resources available in your community.

In the secondary mode, there is still no indication of a specific terrorist plan to attack your community. In this mode, there is still a good chance that the predicted hurricane will swing far south of your community. In the secondary mode though, your perception of likelihood is higher.

What should your fire service organization do if DHS raises the HSAS from yellow to orange for the financial sector in specific cities? What if there is a theft in your area of uniforms or vehicles that would allow access to restricted areas? In such circumstances, fire service personnel may need to maintain a heightened level of operational security and remain alert to behavior by any visitors or service providers that seem suspect. The following represent a brief overview of **potential intervention activities appropriate to the Secondary Mode:**

- Report any activities that might indicate surveillance of fire operations.
- Maintain contact with the Local Emergency Planning Committee (LEPC) or an equivalent organization.
- Maintain daily contact with law enforcement or the appropriate counterterrorism point of contact, and enact "be on the lookout" (BOLO) operations at all key sites.
- Search all bags, cases and parcels, including those carried by employees.
- Screen all incoming postal and electronic mail, phone calls, deliveries, and visitors.
- Secure all facilities, apparatus, and equipment, including access to computer networks.
- Review all threat analysis and vulnerability assessments for department critical infrastructure, implementing countermeasures where needed.
- Maintain a high level of communication with all staff and mandate review of all special operations and terrorism plans.
- Request police patrol of apparatus located away from fire stations.
- Vary operational routines, such as response routes or command post locations, making sure to avoid predictability.
- Maintain communication with private sector organizations, especially vendors, to ensure critical equipment and resources remain available (communications, fuel, vehicles, etc.).
- Inspect facility exteriors on a regular but unpredictable basis.
- Place on-call and off-call Emergency Operations Center teams on alert.

(*Fire and Emergency Services Preparedness Guide…*; and Martinez)

In the aftermath of Katrina, the New Orleans Fire Department lost 23 of 33 fire stations. But core departmental capabilities were preserved because prior to the storm many of the most vulnerable stations were abandoned. Equipment and personnel were redeployed to higher ground in accordance with preexisting plans. According to the *Times-Picayune*, "Twenty-three engines, nine ladder trucks, five squirts and 27 water tankers, along with the dozens of firefighters who use them, have been redeployed to the remaining stations and the six makeshift locations." (Philbin)

Because the perception of risk is higher, there is often a greater motivation to reduce risk when your community enters the secondary mode. There have been alerts of an increased risk from an intentional threat to a specific target category. Mass transit systems and financial institutions have been among the terrorist targets identified. In the secondary mode—or phase—it is typical to increase protective measures related to specific target categories. Secondary mode decisions are aimed at reducing a more specific risk through protection, deterrence, or preemption.

In the secondary mode, your community may choose to **shift attention from one set of risk priorities to a different set of risk priorities**. For example, through the collaborative process outlined previously your community may determine that a natural threat —perhaps an earthquake—is the potential catastrophe that should be your priority during primary mode. As long as your strategic intelligence and analysis suggests that no threat is in the secondary or tertiary mode, then your priority is to mitigate the catastrophic threat of an earthquake.

However, when strategic intelligence and analysis indicates that a natural, accidental, or intentional threat has reached secondary mode you may want to shift at least some of your assets to protect, deter, and preempt the emerging risk. Consider the relationship between tsunamis and earthquakes. When an earthquake registers off the west coast, the potentially catastrophic event poses its own cascading, or secondary, threat since a magnitude 6.7 earthquake, or stronger, is often accompanied by a tsunami. Therefore, an earthquake off the coast raises the risk of a tsunami and leads to heightened awareness of the potential, though not certain, need to evacuate coastal areas.

In most communities, the level of response depends on the perceived level of vulnerability. The response may also reflect the perceived "price" of responding. To protect, deter, or preempt a risk that is at the secondary mode disrupts normal operations. The price is more likely to be acceptable when decision-makers define risks through a collaborative process of information sharing, threat recognition, and managing risk.

If your intelligence and analysis indicate a secondary mode *catastrophic* risk, this is the most important decision-making and action phase. You should do everything possible to prevent or mitigate a potential catastrophe prior to a risk entering the tertiary mode.

Some communities activate Incident Command Centers at this point, forward deploy emergency supplies, and evacuate or prepare high-risk populations (such as the elderly or ill) for evacuation. Many of these tasks involve fire service personnel.

When the risk of flooding reaches the secondary mode sandbagging usually begins. When the risk of wildfire reaches the secondary mode outdoors burning and fireworks are usually banned. When life-threatening heat waves are predicted, the locations of emergency cooling centers are announced and public-service messages begin to prepare

Characteristics of Primary and Secondary Modes

PRIMARY	SECONDARY
• No specific threat identified	• No specific threat identified
	• Threat capability identified that is relevant to local situation
• No unusual vulnerability known	• Threat capability exposes local vulnerability
• Likelihood of risk considered low	• Likelihood of risk increases

What are the signs and symptoms of a risk entering the **tertiary mode**?

How will you recognize and measure these signs and symptoms?

How will you communicate the shift into tertiary mode?

How will you think through and plan operational adjustments to an emerging risk?

the community for what's ahead. It is during the secondary mode that communities in the path of a possible hurricane tape and board windows and take other protective measures.

Public communication is a major element in the secondary mode. Effective public communication deters—maybe even preempts—many of the most troublesome public reactions to an emerging risk. The principles of TALK (see page 47) are important to build into your intervention decision. In the secondary mode, there is enough of a recognized risk to motivate attention and there is still time for the public to respond positively to what they are being told.

In many ways both the primary and secondary modes are focused on **making good use of time available to prevent and mitigate**, rather than just respond to risk.

In March 2004, British law enforcement arrested eight suspected terrorists, seizing a half-ton of the same fertilizer used to make bombs in Istanbul, Bali, and Oklahoma City. The arrests were the result of communication intercepts monitored months earlier. After initial surveillance, investigators decided the plotters were still in the process of gathering bomb elements. The risk was still in the secondary mode. As a result, surveillance continued in order to identify all the plotters, their sources of support, and other operational details. The arrest was timed to ensure the risk did not enter the tertiary mode, but it

was delayed to maximize the options available in the secondary mode.

In many cases, a risk in the secondary mode will "blow over" (sometimes literally). In other cases the redeployment of assets to protect, deter, or preempt will contribute to the risk being reduced, delayed, or prevented. Recognizing when a serious risk is emerging gives your community more options—and often more time—to reduce the risk before it is too late.

TERTIARY MODE: PROTECT, DETER, AND PREEMPT

When a risk enters the tertiary mode **it is almost too late**. Some argue that when a tertiary risk emerges you can respond, but it is past time to prevent.

Fire Captain Larry Collins of the Los Angeles County Fire Department explains how firefighters can recognize a Tertiary Threat while engaged in routine activities. On April 29, 1997 a dispatch sent the USAR company Collins commanded to rescue an unconscious woman on the beach. The person was lying on the beach under a cliff and while Collins' company responded to the incident they discovered an Igloo cooler with wires protruding. The cooler contained a bomb. Collins summarizes the significance of the incident as follows:

...this technical rescue operation-cum-mystery and terrorist threat is archetypal of a seemingly benign situation that ultimately reveals a nature and hazards quite different from those suspected from the first outward appearances: a seemingly 'innocent' rescue that very nearly turned deadly for unsuspecting firefighters and emergency room staff. (*Rescue and Terrorism...*, p. 94)

In the tertiary mode, **a threat *capability* has morphed into a *specific* threat**—or something very close to a specific threat. You have a serious heart problem, your community is dead center in the hurricane landfall zone, a truck carrying toxic chemicals is missing, or terrorists have targeted your community for attack.

As early as possible in the tertiary mode is when voluntary evacuations of the secondary mode become mandatory evacuations. This is when a massive police presence may deter a terrorist attack and increase the possibility of preempting a terrorist attack. In the tertiary mode, first responders are already at or on their way to the scene of the incident.

The U.S. air transportation system and nuclear industry operate in the tertiary mode most of the time. Massive resources are deployed to protect against, deter, and preempt natural, accidental, and intentional threats to recognized vulnerabilities. The risk is considered very likely. The potential consequences are considered devastating. As a result, the investment in managing the tertiary risk is enormous.

What are the signs and symptoms of a risk entering the tertiary mode? How will you recognize and measure these signs and symptoms? How will you communicate the shift into tertiary mode? How will you think through and plan operational adjustments to an emerging risk?

The following activities are among the **types of intervention decisions appropriate to protecting fire service capabilities in response to a Tertiary Mode threat.**

- Provided no attacks occur in your jurisdiction, or in jurisdictions where mutual aid is required, review your threat analysis and vulnerability assessments to determine what targets similar to those attacked are within your jurisdiction or mutual aid agreements.
- Maintain contact with law enforcement or appropriate counterterrorism points of contact on a daily basis, or more frequently if the situation requires.
- Prepare to provide short-term housing to employees and their families.
- Prepare to implement continuity of operations plans.
- Close and secure all unnecessary facilities, setting alarms where installed.
- Close any departmental underground parking garages to incoming traffic.
- Consider releasing all non-critical personnel.
- Notify special teams as needed, e.g. urban area search and rescue.
- Keep all apparatus and active duty staff in quarters except during response.
- Arrange with law enforcement to close access to any areas where response to an incident is required.

(*Fire and Emergency Services Preparedness Guide...*; and Martinez)

🔵 On your CD please see *Incident Management and Emergency Management* by Sauter and Carafano for key action elements that begin to move from tertiary prevention to primary response.

Characteristics of Secondary and Tertiary Modes

SECONDARY
- No specific threat identified
- Threat capability identified that is relevant to local situation
- Threat capability exposes local vulnerability
- Likelihood of risk increases

TERTIARY
- Specific threat identified
- Local vulnerability to the threat exists
- Likelihood of risk is considered high

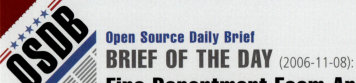

Open Source Daily Brief
BRIEF OF THE DAY (2006-11-08):
Fire Department Foam Approved to Fight Avian Flu

Biological threats such as pandemic influenza, anthrax, plague, and food contamination are difficult to prevent. The nature of the threat, whether natural, accidental, or intentional, makes little difference in managing its risk. Effective surveillance and quick action to contain an outbreak mitigates the risk from these threats.

The poultry industry has never attempted to prepare for a bird sickness that threatens humans. An outbreak of avian flu did occur in Delaware, in February 2004, and a month later spread to Maryland. It was not the H5N1 strain. In the case of animal influenza, extermination is usually the best way to protect both animal and human health. The traditional method of poultry extermination uses carbon dioxide gas. Implementation of the gas method requires up to 15 specially trained personnel.

The University of Delaware recently tested and confirmed a faster and less expensive method for the extermination of poultry populations in the case of an epidemic threat. The same sort of foam fire departments use to suppress fires eliminates an infected population through mass suffocation. With modest training, as few as two personnel deployed the foam method in a test environment.

The more quickly a contagious population is contained the less likely other animal populations are threatened and the risk of animal to human transmission minimized. Use of fire suppression foam is an easier, quicker, and less expensive method. The state of Delaware, with one of the nation's largest commercial poultry populations, plans to invest in its own foam application technology.

Many current fire department platforms carry five-gallon foam application containers. However, larger application units are unusual outside the aviation and chemical sectors. Much larger application containers are required for avian control purposes. Even where the technology is available, authorities need to address issues of jurisdictional authority and finances in advance through mutual aid agreements. Use of commercial assets —such as a fire suppression unit owned by a private chemical company—also require working out in advance. Effective mitigation results from a very rapid response.

PREVENTION RELEVANCE:
Early and effective mitigation of a pandemic threat—whether the source is natural, accidental, or intentional—is fundamental to prevention and preparedness.

PREVENTION TECHNIQUES:
- Identify innovative methods of prevention and mitigation.
- Inventory available assets.
- Ensure training and exercising to be prepared.

PREVENTION THOUGHT: Risk Management
Birds and swine are the principal animal incubators of pandemic influenza.

Do you live in an area with significant populations of birds or swine?

Are the first responders in your area prepared to contain and control animal incubators of diseases such as avian flu?

The Open Source Daily Brief is a service of the Institute for Preventive Strategies (©IPS). You can register to receive the OSDBs at www.preventivestrategies.net.

MAKING AN EFFECTIVE DECISION

We noted in Chapter 5 that selecting a community's risk priorities is often contentious. To overcome this contentiousness it was emphasized that the decision should involve all the preparedness professions.

The risk priorities your community selects also serve as the focus of the decision to intervene. The decision must specify what to do and when. Unless you complement priorities with a practical plan for what and when to act, the priority is like a skeleton without muscle: it falls apart.

As the quick consideration of primary, secondary, and tertiary modes suggests, this decision must reflect several different possibilities. The decision must also encompass a variety of responses by many of the preparedness professions.

Peter Drucker, one of the great strategists of the last century, wrote "The understanding that underlies the right decision grows out of the clash and conflict of divergent opinions and out of the serious consideration of competing alternatives... **The first rule is to make sure that everyone who will have to do something to make the decision effective—or who could sabotage it—has been forced to participate responsibly in the discussion.** This is not 'democracy.' It is salesmanship." (*Management: Tasks, Responsibilities, Practices*)

Collaboration in information sharing leads to collaboration in threat recognition. Collaboration in threat recognition is the foundation for a shared understanding of risk and the choice of a common risk priority or set of risk priorities. A shared commitment to a risk priority is necessary to develop a shared understanding of how the decision regarding that priority will be translated into action.

Drucker continues, "Converting a decision into action requires answering several distinct questions:

'Who has to know of this decision?'

'What action has to be taken?'

'Who is to take it?'

'And what does the action have to be so that the people who have to do it can do it?'

The first and last of these are too often overlooked—with dire results."

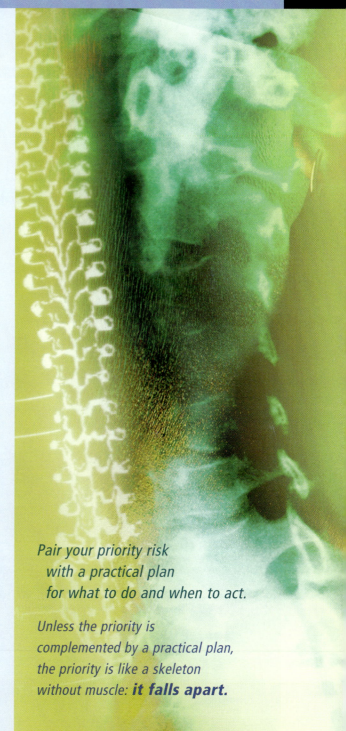

Pair your priority risk with a practical plan for what to do and when to act.

Unless the priority is complemented by a practical plan, the priority is like a skeleton without muscle: **it falls apart.**

A Real Decision (a decision that is ready to be implemented) according to Peter Drucker answers four questions:

1. Who has to know of this decision?
2. What action has to be taken?
3. Who is to take it?
4. What does the action have to be so that the people who have to do it can do it?

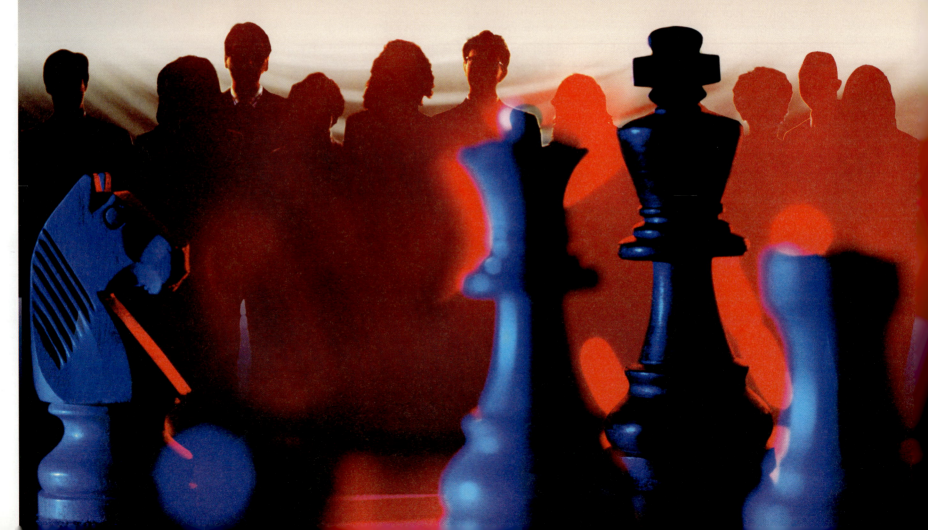

While your community may not yet have a fully collaborative process of information sharing, threat recognition, and risk management, do your best to answer the following questions based on what you currently perceive.

What is your community's **risk priority**?

_____
_____
_____

Is this priority a potential **catastrophic** risk?

yes   no

If no, is your community giving any priority to a catastrophic risk?

yes   no

If no, why not?

_____
_____
_____

If yes, what is your **highest priority** catastrophic risk?

_____
_____
_____

If your community has identified a catastrophic risk priority, please answer the following questions in regard to that risk. Otherwise, please answer the following questions for your community's highest **non-catastrophic** risk priority.

Is this risk priority currently in the
❑ **Primary Mode**
❑ **Secondary Mode**
❑ **Tertiary Mode** *(If so, stop filling out this form and try to stop the risk from growing!)*

What is currently being done to **protect** against the priority risk?

_____
_____
_____
_____

Which preparedness professions are involved in **protection**?

_____
_____
_____
_____

What is currently being done to **deter** the risk?

_____
_____
_____
_____

Which preparedness professions are involved in **deterrence**?

_____
_____
_____
_____

What is currently being done to **preempt** the risk?

_____
_____
_____
_____

Which preparedness professions are involved in **preemption**?

_____
_____
_____
_____

Were any of the preparedness professions identified above NOT involved in selecting the risk priority?

yes   no

If so, which ones?

_____
_____
_____
_____

If some of the preparedness professions involved in implementing the risk priority were excluded from its selection, what has been done to ensure understanding of and support for the risk priority?

_____
_____
_____
_____

More Communications or Shared Purposes?

The most common criticism of any management system—by far—is "poor communications." In almost every organization the most common complaint is that "my manager does not communicate with me enough" or "I don't understand what I am supposed to be doing" or "the direction I receive is inconsistent and contradictory." Organizational surveys almost always produce a call for more communication between managers and employees.

In many organizations a careful follow-up study of these complaints has found a wealth of information and communication, but the absence of a shared understanding of purpose or a mutually recognized set of goals. When this is the case the solution is not so much "more" communication as "better" communication.

In most organizations communications are misunderstood because the sender and receiver do not share a common context. Managers usually intend their tactical communications to be heard in the context of previously discussed strategic objectives and goals. Those receiving the tactical communications do not always make the strategic connection.

This is especially the case when the receiver has not been involved in crafting the strategic objectives and goals. Managers have an obligation to regularly communicate strategy. Those receiving management communications have an obligation to give attention to strategy and to ask questions about strategy.

Effective human networks absolutely depend on a shared understanding of strategy.

Your responses to the questions on the previous page go a long way to answering three of Drucker's four action questions: "Who has to know of this decision?" "What action has to be taken?" "Who is to take it?"

Drucker makes the point that in most organizations when these three questions have been answered, most managers perceive the decision has been made. He insists that this is wrong. Drucker contends the decision to intervene is still unfinished. There is still one more very important question to answer.

"And what does the action have to be so that the people who have to do it can do it?" Perhaps easier: **What capacities are necessary in the people who have to carry out the decision?**

In preventing catastrophe, this is largely a matter of staffing, training, and equipping. **Are there enough people with sufficient skills and the right tools to do the job?**

Do you have trained intelligence analysts?

Do you have basic information sharing tools?

Do you have the resources necessary to bring together preparedness professionals from across your region to develop the collaborative processes needed to implement the prevention cube?

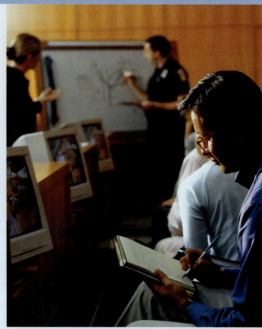
Source: iStockphoto

Do you have the resources to train and exercise together using the scenarios that are most appropriate to your community?

Do you have the resources to provide each of your preparedness professions with the equipment they need to prevent catastrophe?

What Drucker's fourth question also implies is that action has to be designed to reflect the reality of those who are to do it. For example, preventing catastrophe requires collaboration. Collaboration is tough. Collaboration takes time and energy. Do not try to prevent catastrophe unless you are willing to invest in collaboration. Do not ask people to do the impossible.

PLANNING AND RESOURCING

In the 2006 federal budget, more than $1.7 billion was appropriated for Homeland Security grants to states and localities. These monies are committed by Congress to assist your community and region to do your best to prevent catastrophe.

There are perpetual controversies about how this money is distributed. Any time billions of dollars are distributed there will be ongoing debate about the criteria and processes for deciding what money goes where. In any program of this size there will be mistakes of judgment and procedure.

But the common goal is to direct more money to those communities and regions with the highest risk and the most effective plan for managing the risk.

According to the Department of Homeland Security, "In fiscal year 2006, DHS adopted a risk and effectiveness-based approach to allocating funding for certain programs within (the Homeland Security Grant Program) HSGP. This approach aligns federal resources with national priorities and target capabilities established by the Interim National Preparedness Goal to generate the highest return on investment in increasing the nation's level of preparedness."

The principled process of decision-making represented by the prevention cube provides each community and region with a realistic definition of potential risks. It puts in place a collaborative process for making sound risk management decisions. These outcomes enhance the ability of your community to meet the risk and effectiveness criteria by which federal grants are awarded.

Beginning in 2006, those applying for federal Homeland Security Grants were required to complete an "Investment Justification." The investment justification is another way of asking Drucker's four action questions. **Following are most of the issues posed by the DHS Investment Justification process:**

- Explain how the State/Urban Area is organizing to implement this investment over the identified geographic area(s).

- Discuss the collaboration process you have, or will establish, with other regions and jurisdictions (inter- and intra-State) within or beyond the geographic/demographic area of this investment. Discuss when and how you will engage stakeholders from those regions in specific support for this investment.

- Discuss anticipated impacts of this investment and how the requested funding will help attain/achieve expected impacts. Consider the population and areas affected, and other entities (jurisdictions, disciplines) that could leverage the outcomes and impacts of the solution presented by this investment.

- Discuss how the implementation of this investment will decrease or mitigate risk.

- Describe what the potential Homeland Security risks of not funding this investment are.

- Identify potential challenges to the effective implementation of this investment (e.g. stakeholder buy-in, sustainability, aggressive timelines).

- Explain how the identified challenge will be addressed and mitigated.

- Describe the management team, including roles and responsibilities, that will be accountable for the oversight and implementation of this investment, and the overall management approach they will apply for the implementation of this investment.

- Discuss funding resources beyond FY2006 HSGP that have been identified and will be leveraged to support the implementation and sustainment of this investment.

- Provide a high level timeline, including milestones and dates, for the implementation of this investment. Possible areas for inclusion are stakeholder engagement, planning, major acquisition/purchases, training, exercises, and process/policy updates.

(The complete *DHS Investment Justification User's Guide* is available on your CD.)

CHAPTER 6 — DECIDE TO INTERVENE

Poor Planning Increases Vulnerability

In June 2006 the Department of Homeland Security completed a national review of over 2700 emergency operation plans and supportive documents. **The top three findings were:**

1. The majority of the Nation's current emergency operations plans and planning processes cannot be characterized as fully adequate, feasible, or acceptable to manage catastrophic events as defined in the National Response Plan (NRP).

2. States and urban areas are not conducting adequate collaborative planning as a part of "steady state" preparedness.

3. Assumptions in Basic Plans do not adequately address catastrophic events.

Looking ahead, the DHS report notes:

"When a catastrophic event overwhelms a single jurisdiction or has region-wide impact, effective response hinges on combined action and pooling of resources… Combined planning represents the single convergence point where Federal, State, and local concepts and resources can be translated into specific patterns of action and synchronized to achieve unity of effort… The initial conclusions in this Report reflect an understanding that planning is a quest, not a guarantee. Even the best planners cannot fully anticipate surprise or novelty, or compensate for poor incident management. While no plan can guarantee success, inadequate plans are proven contributors to failure."

A complete copy of the Nationwide Plan Review is available on your CD.

The Department of Homeland Security specifically invites applications for grants related to Personnel, Planning, Organization, Equipment, Training, and Exercises.

DHS gives particular attention to Investment Justifications that advance National Priorities and Target Capabilities. These are specified in the National Preparedness Goal (this is available on your CD) and related documents. But the principal criteria for receiving federal support are the clear identification of risk—especially catastrophic risk—and the presentation of an effective plan for responding to that risk.

The more thorough your analysis and presentation of risk and the more complete and credible your plan for managing the risk,

the more likely your community will maximize its federal support.

Too often, answering these questions is left to grant writers. For meaningful answers—for answers that result in practical action—the questions must be asked at the operational and strategic level for all the preparedness professions.

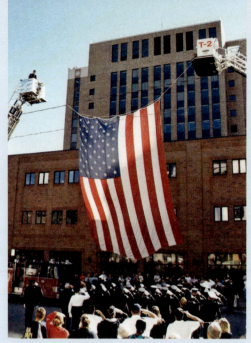

Bloomington Fire Department 9-11 Memorial Service, Bloomington, IL

These are questions for the entire community. These are questions and answers for the firefighter, the fire captain, and the fire chief.

PREPARING FOR CATASTROPHE

It is said that when others are concerned about "doing things right," the leader focuses on **"doing the right thing."** Choosing the right thing can be tough. Faced with an abundance of natural, accidental, and intentional threats, choosing the right focus is a significant challenge. Failure to make a choice is a dereliction of duty.

To be a leader is to make a decision. To be an effective leader the choice should be made in a clear and principled way. An effective leader involves others in choosing to ensure shared understanding of each choice.

A good leader is always aware of risk. The leader works to understand, prevent, and mitigate risk, but a good leader avoids the temptation to minimize risk. A real leader is ready to keep the reality of risk at the forefront of everyone's thinking and doing.

The greater the risk, the more the leader focuses on the risk. Scan for it, analyze it, respond to it, and assess your scanning, analyzing, and responding. Change your choices based on new information, but don't avoid choosing. Only by making self-aware choices do you have any chance of effectively managing the risk to you, your colleagues, and your community.

Some have said that the greatest risk we face—especially in dealing with the terrorist threat—**is the loss of freedom**. If so, with every conscious and principled choice we mitigate that risk.

Source: iStockphoto

"Freedom is not merely the opportunity to do as one pleases;

neither is it merely the opportunity to choose between set alternatives.

Freedom is, first of all, the chance to formulate the available choices,

to argue over them —

and then, the opportunity to choose."

—C. WRIGHT MILLS

DECIDE TO INTERVENE:
Chapter Review

Define the nature of a risk appropriate for **primary mode intervention**.

Define the nature of a risk appropriate for **secondary mode intervention**.

Define the nature of a risk that requires **tertiary mode intervention**.

Give an example of primary mode **protection**.

Give an example of secondary mode **protection**.

Peter Drucker has said an effective decision answers four questions. In your own words what are these key questions?

1

Give an example of primary mode **deterrence**.

Give an example of secondary mode **deterrence**.

2

3

Give an example of primary mode **preemption**.

Give an example of secondary mode **preemption**.

4

CHAPTER 6 — DECIDE TO INTERVENE

APPLY WHAT YOU HAVE LEARNED

Use your CD to access the Intervention Advanced Exercise. Select the **Chapter 6** Certificate Course link located in the Online Exercises section of your CD.

In the role of a Senior Captain in the San Luis Rey® Fire Department you are eager to apply what you and your collaboration team have learned about the threat by developing an intervention plan.

It is now about 3 weeks before the date of the planned attack. The San Luis Rey Fire Department has been on the lookout for suspicious activity such as unusual interest in or surveillance of key San Luis Rey targets by non-officials. This resulted in the arrest of one of the key terrorists.

Was this enough to dissuade the other terrorists from carrying out their primary plan? Is the risk diminished? Does this impact your decision to intervene? Who should be involved in the decision to intervene?

Three San Luis Rey Senior Fire Captains will provide their views on intervention. Given the nature of the threat, vulnerabilities, consequences, and resulting risks, which intervention plan has the best chance of succeeding?

Note: If you have already enrolled in the Homeland Security Terrorism Prevention Certificate Course for Fire Service Professionals (©IPS) you can go directly to the exercise by using the Online Exercises Direct Access links on your CD or by typing this URL into your browser's address window:

www.preventivestrategies.net/go/mhfs-adv-ex-intervene

For first time access, use this initial URL:
www.preventivestrategies.net/go/mhfs-enroll

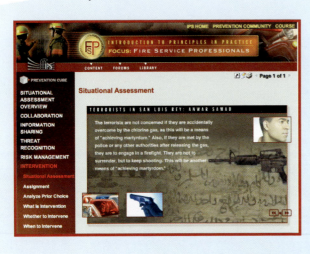

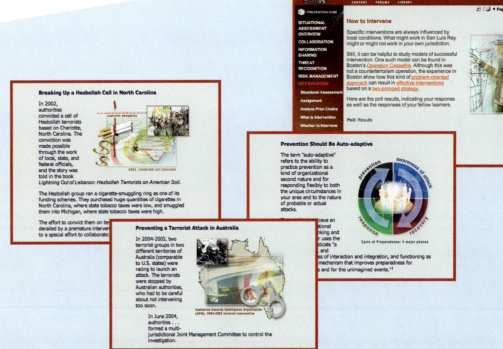

San Luis Rey® is a fictional jurisdiction designed by Teleologic Learning LLC.
All characters, locations, and events are fictitious and intended for instructional purposes only.

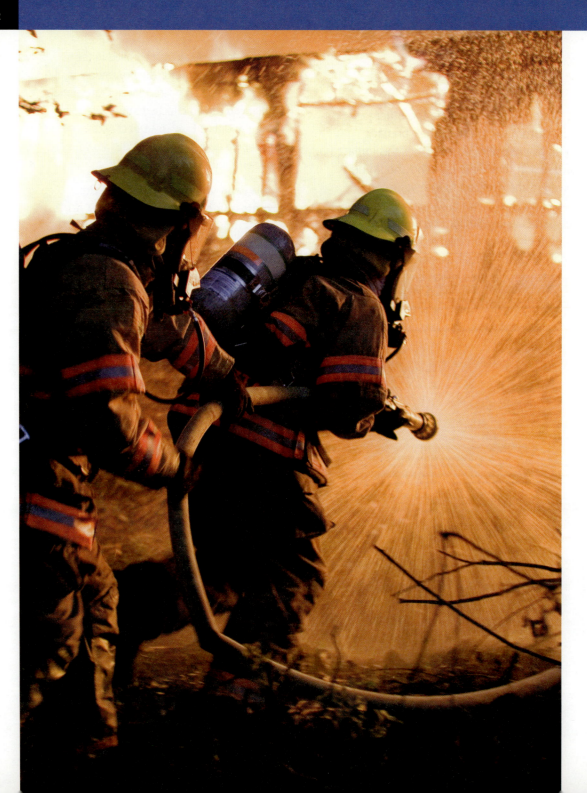

ACKNOWLEDGMENTS

Catastrophe Preparation and Prevention for Fire Service Professionals

Principal Authors: CDR Craig Baldwin USN (Ret), Larry R. Irons PhD, and Philip J. Palin

Principal Learning Architects: Philip J. Palin and Kari Sandhaas

The principles of prevention on which this workbook is based originated with William V. Pelfrey, PhD. The prevention cube is a tool by which these principles may be practiced. The prevention cube was conceived by Christopher Bellavita, Philip Palin, and William Pelfrey.

The authors are pleased to acknowledge specific contributions to this publication by Sheri Chirco, Angela Cox, Robert Halprin, Jason Kirchgessner, Aaron Kruger, Jill Miller, Steve Newton, Peggy Payne, William Thomas, Mark Tovey, and Shannon Widmer.

Particular acknowledgement is due John Bowen who has served as the principal architect and editor of the resource CD which accompanies this workbook.

Recognition and gratitude are owed to the following organizations and individuals for photos, photo research assistance, and permissions: Keith Ranney and Eric Vaughn, Bloomington Fire Department, Bloomington, IL; Jerry McCay, Sangamon County Rescue Squad, New Berlin, IL.

The authors benefited from advice and reviews by Christopher Bellavita, Garry Briese, Darrell Darnell, Luis A. Guzman, and William Pelfrey.

The authors appreciate the support and guidance of McGraw-Hill in developing this series, with special thanks to David Culverwell, Elizabeth Haefele, Jim Kelly, Claire Merrick, Linda Schreiber, Richard Weimer, and Sarah Wood.

The McGraw Hill Companies engaged Teleologic Learning Company (www.teleologic.net) to develop the learning architecture for the Catastrophe Preparation series.

San Luis Rey is a registered service mark of Teleologic Learning LLC.

AUTHOR PROFILES

Craig Baldwin is a retired naval officer with experience in space systems, intelligence, and tactical operations. Mr. Baldwin consults on Homeland Security issues for Teleologic Learning Company and is a Senior Fellow with the National Institute for Strategic Preparedness.

Larry Irons completed his PhD from Washington University. He is a Senior Fellow with the National Institute for Strategic Preparedness and the principal author of *Open Source Daily Brief*.

Philip Palin is the Chief Executive Officer of Teleologic Learning Company. He is a consultant on strategy and learning to several public and private sector organizations. Mr. Palin is also a Senior Fellow with the National Institute for Strategic Preparedness.

ACKNOWLEDGMENTS

The McGraw-Hill Companies appreciates the following individuals who reviewed and offered their advice on *Catastrophe Preparation and Prevention for Fire Service Professionals.*

Trent M. Atkins, PEM, EFO, CFOD
    Lansing Fire Department
    Lansing, Michigan

Don Beckering
    Minnesota State Colleges and Universities
    St. Paul, Minnesota

Tom Bentley
    John Wood Community College
    Quincy, Illinois

Gregory M. Brown
    Eureka Fire Protection District
    Eureka, Missouri

Dennis Childress
    Orange County Fire Authority
    San Clemente, California

Kenneth E. Crews
    Durham Fire Department
    Durham, North Carolina

Gregg S. Dawson
    North Central TX Council of Governments
    Arlington, Texas

Ron Deadman
    Avondale Fire-Rescue
    Avondale, Arizona

David K. Donohue, MA, EMT-P
    Shepherdstown Fire Department
    Shepherdstown, West Virginia

David W. Lewis
    University of Maryland, Maryland Fire
    & Rescue Institute
    College Park, Maryland

Murrey E. Loflin
    West Virginia University Fire Service Extension
    Morgantown, West Virginia

Stephen S. Malley
    Department Chair of Public Safety—
    Weatherford College
    Weatherford, Texas

Al Martinez, Fire Chief, Steger Fire Department
    Prairie State College
    Chicago Heights, Illinois

John A. McCoy
    Emergency Incident Consultants
    Fayetteville, North Carolina

Philip J. Oakes
    Laramie County Fire District # 6
    Burns, Wyoming

James L. Paturas, CEM, EMTP, CHS-IV, FACCP
    Yale New Haven Center for Emergency
    Preparedness and Disaster Response
    New Haven, Connecticut

Keith Richter
    Contra Costa County Fire Dist.
    Pleasant Hill, California

Richard Shoaf
    STCI
    Lake Saint Louis, Missouri

Karl K. Thompson
    Tennessee Fire and Codes Academy
    Bell Buckle, Tennessee

Bruce Trego
    Office of the State Fire Commissioner
    Lewistown, Pennsylvania

Ed Vasques, Assistant Chief
    Sacramento Fire Department,
    Special Operations Division
    Sacramento, California

Douglas R. Williams
    US Fire Administration—National Fire
    Academy
    Emmitsburg, Maryland

Thomas J. Wutz
    New York State Office of Fire Prevention
    and Control
    Albany, New York

WORKS CITED

in *Catastrophe Preparation and Prevention for Fire Service Professionals*

Many readers using this workbook will find it helpful to extend their study to include three other texts:

- *Homeland Security: A Complete Guide to Understanding, Preventing, and Surviving Terrorism* by Mark Sauter and James Jay Carafano.

- *Terrorism and Counterterrorism Understanding the New Security Environment, Readings and Interpretations.* Eds. Russell D. Howard and Reid L. Sawyer.

- *The McGraw-Hill Homeland Security Handbook.* Ed. David G. Kamien.

Studied together these resources offer a rigorous review of strategic, operational, and tactical issues related to many core issues of Homeland Security.

Works below are listed in alphabetical order.

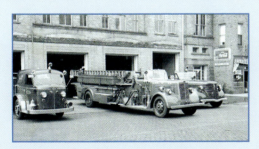

Central Fire Station, 1940s.
Bloomington Fire Department, Bloomington, IL

Agner, Jon P. "Got Clearance?" *Fire Management Today* 64:4, Fall 2004, p. 12.

"Apex Facility Fire Prevention Shortcomings," *HazMat Magazine*. November 6, 2006.

Arquilla, John, Dave Ronfeldt, and Michele Zanini. "Networks, Netwar, and Information-Age Terrorism." *Terrorism and Counterterrorism: Understanding the New Security Environment, Readings and Interpretations*, Eds. Russell D. Howard and Reid L. Sawyer. McGraw-Hill, 2004.

Bachman, Eric G. "Preincident Intelligence of Quarries." *Fire Engineering* 158:11, November 2005, pp. 87-91.

Bachman, Eric G. "Water Supply Preincident Intelligence," *Fire Engineering* 158:11, November 2005, pp. 95-105.

Bazerman, Max, and Michael Watkins. *Predictable Surprises: The Disasters You Should Have Seen Coming, and How to Prevent Them*. Harvard Business School Press, 2004.

Bigley, Gregory A. and Karlene H. Roberts. "The Incident Command System: High-Reliability Organizing for Complex and Volatile Task Environments." *Academy of Management Journal* 44:6, December 2001, pp. 1281-1299.

WORKS CITED

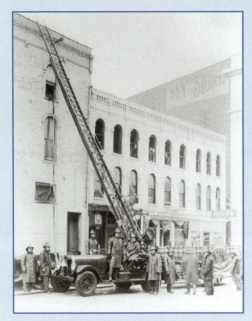

1916 ladder truck.
Bloomington Fire Department, Bloomington, IL

Bonner, Lynn. "State Toughens Hazardous Waste Rules." *The News & Observer*, June 27, 2007.

CARVER Plus Shock Method for Food Sector Vulnerability Assessments. Available online at: http://www.ngfa.org/pdfs/Carver_Shock_Primer.pdf

Chemical Emergency Preparedness and Prevention. U.S. Environmental Protection Agency. Available online at: http://yosemite.epa.gov/oswer/ceppoweb.nsf/content/ChemicalsInYourCommunity.htm?OpenDocument#lepc

Cilluffo, Frank, et al. *Defending America in the 21st Century: New Challenges, New Organizations, and New Policies*. Center for Strategic and International Studies, December 2000.

Coleman, David, quoted by Bill Roberts. "Making Beautiful Music: Culture change, not technology, is key to collaboration." *CIO Magazine*, December 15, 1999–January 1, 2000.

Coleman, Toby. "Apex Wants Full Hazmat Disclosure." *The News & Observer*, October 25, 2006. Available online at: http://www.newsobserver.com/1360/story/502585.html

Collins, Larry. "Rescue and Terrorism, Part 1." *Fire Engineering* 156:8, August 2003, pp. 87-94.

Conetta, Carl. "Dislocating Alcyoneus: How to combat al-Qaeda and the new terrorism." *Project on Defense Alternatives Briefing Memo #23*. Project on Defense Alternatives, June 25, 2002.

Davis, Jack. "Sherman Kent's Final Thoughts on Analyst-Policymaker Relations." *Occasional Papers: Volume 2, Number 3*. The Sherman Kent Center for Intelligence Analysis, June 2003.

DeLisi, Lynn E., Andrea Maurizio, et al. "A Survey of New Yorkers After the Sept. 11, 2001, Terrorist Attacks." *American Journal of Psychiatry*, Vol. 160, 2003.

The Delphi Method: Techniques and Applications. Eds. Harold A. Linstone and Murray Turoff, 2002.

Deonarine, Leonard. "Industrial Terrorism: New Concerns for Fire Departments." *Fire Engineering* 154:1, November 2001, pp. 53-56.

DeVito, Paul, quoted by Tim Logue. "Safe Schools Summit draws 400 officials to Springfield." *Delaware County Daily Times*, March 15, 2006.

Dolnik, Adam. "All God's Poisons: Reevaluating the Threat of Religious Terrorism in Regard to Non-conventional Weapons." *Terrorism and Counterterrorism: Understanding the New Security Environment, Readings and Interpretations*. Eds. Russell D. Howard and Reid L. Sawyer. McGraw-Hill, 2004.

Drucker, Peter. *Management: Tasks, Responsibilities, Practices*. Harper & Row, 1974.

Dynes, Russell R. "Noah and Disaster Planning: The Cultural Significance of the Flood Story." *Journal of Contingencies and Crisis Management* 11:4, December 2005, pp. 170-177.

Felson, Marcus and Ronald V. Clarke. *Opportunity Makes the Thief: Practical Theory for Crime Prevention*. U.K. Home Office, Police and Reducing Crime Unit, 1998.

WORKS CITED

Fire and Emergency Services Preparedness Guide for the Homeland Security Advisory System. FEMA, January 2004. Available online at: http://www.usfa.dhs.gov/downloads/pdf/hsas-guide.pdf

Firewise Programs. Available online at: http://www.firewise.org

Flynn, John P. *Information Management within the New York City Fire Department: Past, Present, and Future.* Masters Thesis. Naval PostGraduate School, 2006. Available online at: http://stinet.dtic.mil/cgi-bin/GetTRDoc?AD=ADA467227&Location=U2&doc=GetTRDoc.pdf

Flynn, Stephen. *The Edge of Disaster.* New York: Random House, 2007.

Foster, Mary. "Under Siege, New Orleans Police Struggle." Associated Press, October 10, 2005.

Franklin, Benjamin. "Protection of Towns from Fire," February 4, 1735 issue of *The Pennsylvania Gazette.* Available online at: http://franklinpapers.org/franklin/framedVolumes.jsp?vol=2&page=012a

Goldsmith, Stephen, and William D. Eggers. *Governing by Network: The New Shape of the Public Sector.* Washington, D.C.: Brookings Institution Press, 2004.

Government Accountability Office. *Combating Nuclear Terrorism: Federal Efforts to Respond to Nuclear and Radiological Threats and to Protect Emergency Response Capabilities Could Be Strengthened.* September 2006. Available online at: http://www.gao.gov/new.items/d061015.pdf

Government Accountability Office. *DHS Is Taking Steps to Enhance Security at Chemical Facilities, but Additional Authority Is Needed.* January 2006.

Harmon, Clarence. "Turning a Popular War into a Populist War: Preparing the American Public for Terrorism." *First to Arrive: State and Local Responses to Terrorism.* Eds. Juliette N. Kayyem and Robyn L. Pangi. Cambridge, MA: MIT Press, 2003.

Hartsoe, Steve. "Aircraft oxygen generators spurred Apex plant fire." *Union-Tribune,* June 27, 2007.

Hashagen, Paul. "Firefighting in Colonial America." *Firehouse Magazine.* Available online at: http://www.firehouse.com/magazine/american/colonial.html

Hawkins, Michelle. "Emergency Planning and Community Right to Know: State Profiles, 1999-2000." National Governors' Association Center for Best Practices, 2000.

Health Physics Society. *Weapon of Mass Destruction Radiological Events.* Available online at: http://hps.org/hsc/documents/wmd_factsheet.pdf

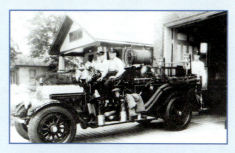

1916 American LaFrance Type 40 Engine. Bloomington Fire Department, Bloomington, IL

Homeland Security Council. *National Planning Scenarios, Version 20.1.* April 2005.

Institute for Preventive Strategies. *Open Source Daily Brief.*

International Association of Chiefs of Police. *Criminal Intelligence Model Policy.* 2003.

Krizan, Lisa. *Intelligence Essentials for Everyone.* Joint Military Intelligence College, June 1999.

Lendrum, Tony. *The Strategic Partnering Pocketbook.* McGraw-Hill, 2004.

LEPC Database. Available online at: http://yosemite.epa.gov/oswer/lepcdb.nsf/HomePage?openForm

Marquis, Kate. "Did 9/11 Matter? Terrorism and Counterterrorism Trends: Past, Present, and Future." *Homeland Security and Terrorism.* Eds. Russell D. Howard, James J.F. Forest, and Joanne Moore. McGraw-Hill, 2005.

WORKS CITED

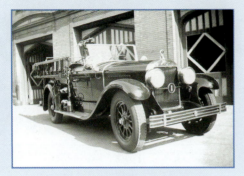

1926 Deluge.
Bloomington Fire Department, Bloomington, IL

Martinez, Brett M. "The Fire Service and Counterterrorism." *Fire Engineering* 159:1, January 2006, pp. 101-106.

Martinez, Brett M. and James M. McLoughlin. "The Fire Service and Counterterrorism: Unified Command." *Fire Engineering* 159:2, February 2006, pp. 73-78.

Mitchell, Earnest, Stephen Doherty, and Bradley C. Hibbard. "Eyes and Ears." *FireChief*, June 1, 2006.

Moore, David T., and Lisa Krizan. "Core Competencies for Intelligence Analysis at the National Security Agency." *Bringing Intelligence About: Practitioners Reflect on Best Practices*. Ed. Russell G. Swenson. Joint Military Intelligence College, Center for Strategic Intelligence Research, 2003.

Moteff, John. *Risk Management and Critical Infrastructure Protection: Assessing, Integrating, and Managing Threats, Vulnerabilities and Consequences*. Congressional Research Service, February 2005.

Moynihan, Donald P. "Leveraging Collaborative Networks in Infrequent Emergency Situations." IBM Center for The Business of Government, June 2005. Available online at: http://www.businessofgovernment.org/pdfs/MoynihanReport.pdf

Murphy, Laura. "Principled Prudence: Civil Liberties and the Homeland Security Practitioner in Post-9/11 America." *The McGraw-Hill Homeland Security Handbook*. Ed. David G. Kamien, 2005.

National Commission on Terrorist Attacks Upon the United States. *The 9/11 Commission Report*. 2004.

National Emergency Management Association. *Model Intrastate Mutual Aid Legislation*. 2004.

National Fire Academy. Available online at: http://www.usfa.dhs.gov/nfa/

New York City Fire Department. *Terrorism and Disaster Preparedness Strategy: Mission Statement of the New York City Fire Department*. 2007. Available online at: http://www.nyc.gov/html/fdny/pdf/events/2007/tdps/terrorism%20strategy_complete.pdf

New York City Fire Department. *Written Statement of the FDNY Before the National Institute of Standards and Technology*. November 22, 2004. Available online at: http://www.nist.gov/public_affairs/ncst/11_22_2004/HaydenStatement_112204.pdf

Office for Domestic Preparedness Guidelines for Homeland Security, Prevention and Deterrence 2003. Department of Homeland Security. Available online at: http://www.ojp.usdoj.gov/odp/docs/ODPPrev1.pdf

Office of Homeland Security. *National Strategy for Homeland Security*. July 2002. Available online at: http://www.whitehouse.gov/homeland/book/nat_strat_hls.pdf

Parachini, John. "Putting WMD Terrorism Into Perspective." *The Washington Quarterly*. Center for Strategic and International Studies, Autumn 2003.

Parnell, Gregory S., Robin Dillon-Merrill, and Terry Bresnick. "Integrating Risk Management with Security and Antiterrorism Resource Allocation Decision Making." *The McGraw-Hill Homeland Security Handbook*. Ed. David G. Kamien. McGraw-Hill, 2005.

Pelfrey, William V. "The Cycle of Preparedness: Establishing a Framework to Prepare for Terrorist Threats." *Journal of Homeland Security and Emergency Management* 2:1, 2005.

Philbin, Walt. "Firefighters Battle Post-Katrina Hurdles." *New Orleans Times-Picayune*, November 21, 2005.

Plaugher, Edward P. "Fire Service Response to Terrorism." *Testimony to the Committee on Commerce, Science, and Technology*. United States Senate. October 11, 2001. Available online at: http://commerce.senate.gov/hearings/101101Plaugher.pdf

Posner, Richard A. *Catastrophe: Risk and Response*. Oxford University Press, 2004.

Preparedness Network (PrepNet). Available online at: http://www.usfa.dhs.gov/training/prepnet/

Robbins, Elizabeth L. "Leadership through Media." *Homeland Security and Terrorism*. Eds. Russell D. Howard, James J.F. Forest, and Joanne Moore. McGraw-Hill, 2005.

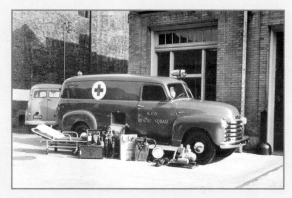

1948 Chevy Squad Car.
Bloomington Fire Department, Bloomington, IL

Rosenzweig, Paul. "Thinking about Civil Liberty and Terrorism." *The McGraw-Hill Homeland Security Handbook*. Ed. David G. Kamien. McGraw-Hill, 2005.

Sackman, Harold. *Delphi Assessment: Expert Opinion, Forecasting, and Group Process*. RAND Corporation, April 1974.

Sauter, Mark, and James Jay Carafano. *Homeland Security: A Complete Guide to Understanding, Preventing, and Surviving Terrorism*. McGraw-Hill, 2005.

Sauter, Mark and James Jay Carafano. "The Mind of a Terrorist: Why They Hate Us." *Homeland Security: A Complete Guide to Understanding, Preventing, and Surviving Terrorism*. McGraw-Hill, 2005.

Sauter, Mark, and James Jay Carafano. "Weapons of Mass Destruction: Understanding the Great Terrorist Threats and Getting Beyond the Hype." *Homeland Security: A Complete Guide to Understanding, Preventing, and Surviving Terrorism*. McGraw-Hill, 2005.

Sesno, Frank. "The Role of Broadcast Media in Homeland Security Communications." *The McGraw-Hill Homeland Security Handbook*. Ed. David G. Kamien. McGraw-Hill, 2005.

Shaw, Sir Eyre Massey. *A Complete Manual of Organization, Machinery, Discipline, and General Working of the Fire Brigade of London*. C & E Leighton, 1876.

Shelley, Craig and Anthony Cole. "Terrorism and Security Issues When Responding to Industrial Facilities." *Fire Engineering* 158:11, November 2005, pp. 63-68.

Stebnicki, Mark. "Psychological Response to Terrorism as an Extraordinary Stressful and Traumatic Life-Event." Public Schools of North Carolina. Available online at: http://www.ncpublicschools.org/safeschools/resources/crisis/national/psychologicalresponse

Stewart, Terry. "Fire Service Risk Management," Public Entity Risk Institute Symposium, 2005. Available online at: http://www.riskinstitute.org/NR/rdonlyres/9B30377C-761C-4142-A67B799AFD542CFE/0/PERI_Symposium_FireServiceRiskMgmt.pdf

Swenson, Russell G. "Introduction." *Bringing Intelligence About: Practitioners Reflect on Best Practices*. Ed. Russell G. Swenson. Joint Military Intelligence College, Center for Strategic Intelligence Research, 2003.

Tucker, Jonathan B. "Historical Trends Related to Bioterrorism: An Empirical Analysis." *Emerging Infectious Diseases* 5:4, July–August 1999.

Tucker, Jonathan B. "Strategies for Countering Terrorism: Lessons from the Israeli Experience." *Journal of Homeland Security*. Homeland Security Institute, March 2003.

USA PATRIOT ACT. Available online at: http://thomas.loc.gov/cgi-bin/query/z?c107:H.R.3162.ENR:

U.S. Army Field Manual 8-285: Treatment of Chemical Agent Casualties and Conventional Military Chemical Injuries. December 1995.

WORKS CITED

U.S. Army Training and Doctrine Command. *A Military Guide to Terrorism in the Twenty-First Century*. August 15, 2005. Available online at: http://www.au.af.mil/au/awc/awcgate/army/guidterr/index.htm

U.S. Department of Homeland Security. *Basic Vulnerability Assessment Worksheet*.

U.S. Department of Homeland Security. *Discussion of the FY 2006 Risk Methodology and the Urban Areas Security Initiative*.

U.S. Department of Homeland Security. *FY 2006 Homeland Security Grant Program: Investment Justification User's Manual*. 2005.

U.S. Department of Homeland Security. *Interim National Preparedness Goal*. March 2005.

U.S. Department of Homeland Security. *National Response Plan*. December 2004. Available online at: http://www.dhs.gov/xlibrary/assets/NRP_FullText.pdf

U.S. Department of Homeland Security. *State and Urban Area Homeland Security Strategy: Guidance on Aligning Strategies with the National Preparedness Goal*. July 2005.

U.S. Department of Justice Bureau of Justice Assistance. *Intelligence Led Policing: The New Intelligence Architecture*. September 2005.

U.S. Department of Justice. *Fusion Center Guidelines: Developing and Sharing Information and Intelligence in a New World, Law Enforcement Intelligence Component*, August 2006. Available online at: http://it.ojp.gov/documents/fusion_center_guidelines_law_enforcement.pdf

U.S. Fire Administration Distance Learning. Available online at: http://www.usfa.dhs.gov/fireservice/training/

U.S. Fire Administration Resources on Fire Safety. Available online at: http://www.usfa.dhs.gov/safety/thisis.shtm

Welch, Alicia L. *Terrorism Awareness and Education as a Prevention Strategy for First Responders*. Masters Thesis. Naval PostGraduate School. 2006. Available online at: http://www.ccc.nps.navy.mil/research/theses/welch06.pdf

White, David. "Industrial STRENGTH." *Fire Chief*, January 1, 2007.

The White House. *National Strategy for Combating Terrorism*. February 2003.

APPENDIX — SAN LUIS REY

SAN LUIS REY®

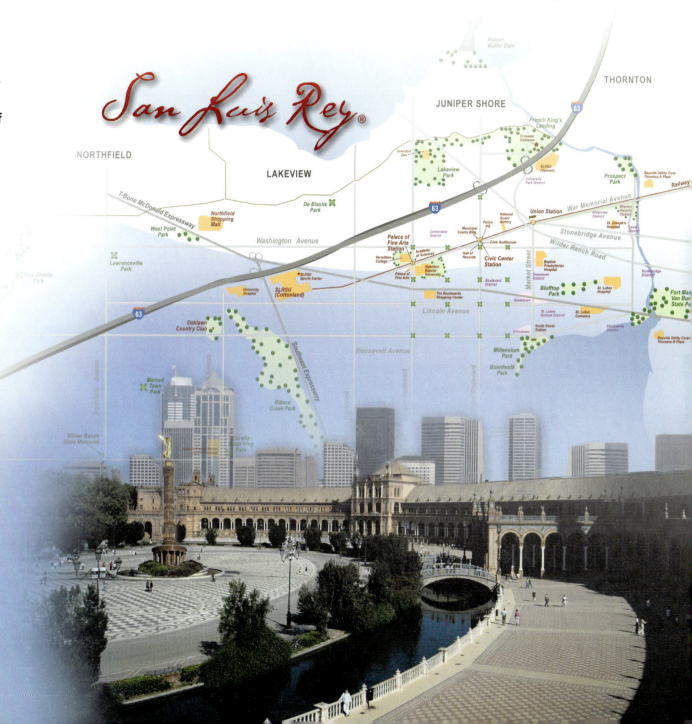

This workbook provides opportunities to apply principles of catastrophe preparedness and prevention utilizing the **fictional jurisdiction of San Luis Rey®**. The online exercises in which you participate all take place in San Luis Rey. Everything you encounter in San Luis Rey is based on **real-world cities, towns, and rural areas**. This is a "practice range" for managing prevention and preparedness problems.

An overview video explaining the fundamentals of San Luis Rey is available on the accompanying CD in the San Luis Rey section. To view this 3 minute video, insert your CD, select **San Luis Rey Information** on the main menu, and then **San Luis Rey — A Strategic Learning Environment**.

A printable PDF fact sheet providing an overview of San Luis Rey facts is also available on the accompanying CD. To view, insert your CD, select **San Luis Rey Information** on the main menu and then **San Luis Rey Facts**.

San Luis Rey® is a registered service mark of Teleologic Learning (LLC).

SAN LUIS REY NEIGHBORHOODS

San Luis Rey is a city of small towns. Since the early days, more than 400 years ago, when the Pueblo de San Luis Rey gathered around the Mission, the place has reflected the needs and hopes of the people who settled here.

The bright white of the Mission, the soft bronze of the Cathedral, the primary colors of the Mercado de Embarcadero define the oldest neighborhood. Below the bluffs, beside the river was the home of the priests and brothers, soldiers and traders, miners, ranchers, and farmers who came to explore and settle this new and mysterious land. The spirit of exploration is at the heart of San Luis Rey.

Today tourists come to explore the roots of the city, and their own roots, in the Spanish Colonial and Native American past. In the blending of these two cultures the new culture of America began. From the solemn Mass of the Assumption, to the rowdy celebration of Mardi Gras, to the beautiful collection of artifacts in the Museum of Indigenous and Folk Art the **Mission District** preserves our memories and the sources of our shared culture. The Mercado, or traditional marketplace,

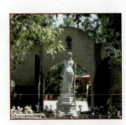

Mission San Luis Rey State Historical Park in the Mission District

winds for four blocks between the ancient adobe and olive trees.

Slightly above the Mission, Cathedral, and Mercado, nestled on a narrow sandstone terrace, is the Convent of Maria del Pilar, famous for its gardens of rosemary and lavender. South along the narrow Avenida de Convento is the late 18th and early 19th century commercial district. Most of the original buildings still stand, including the ornate Perichole Theater built in the 1750s. The Perichole remains a popular venue for opera and chamber music. But across the street a very different sound is produced. The former Cotton Exchange has been converted into a major dance club that has hosted No Doubt, Floetry, Sum41, and other top 40 bands.

The modern influence grows as you walk a few blocks south into the **Canal District**. During the late 19th century warehouses were built along the river and canals were dug to support even more warehouses. This is now a popular neighborhood for artists and musicians. The Surco Center for Contemporary Art shows and sells much of the best work of local artists. The sounds of jazz, rock-and-roll, and new musical styles still being named echo from waterside pubs and clubs that have reclaimed the cavernous buildings. The neighborhood restaurants are as adventurous as the artists and musicians. This is the place to explore what's new and next.

To experience the sure and sophisticated, take a cab or the Presidio Avenue Express Bus to the **Uptown District** for high end shopping and even higher reaching skyscrapers. Gathered around Memorial Circle, Garfield Road, and inside the "Diamond" is what many consider the finest collection of early 20th Century urban architecture anywhere in the world. From the mirrored grandeur of Union Station and the Post Office Building to the soaring pediments of the Board of Trade, Triangle, and Hamilton American buildings you can perceive the energy, ambition, and appreciation for beauty that San Luis Rey has inherited from its founders.

Concerts and fireworks around the Soldier's and Sailor's Column have been a local favorite for nearly a century. In more recent

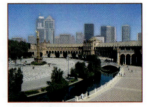

Soldiers and Sailors Circle

years the sidewalks of Memorial Circle have become adorned with al fresco cafes and restaurants. When the trains stopped rolling into Union Station, they were replaced with sophisticated stores carrying exotic goods from around the world. The traditional shopping center of the city along North Market has also been converted into four blocks of pedestrian promenade.

But are you less a consumer and more of a connoisseur? If so, take the Transit Authority subway from the station beneath Memorial Circle four stops west to the Palace of Fine Arts Station (locally know as PFA or Pifa). For most of the first half of the Twentieth Century the wealthiest citizens of San Luis Rey conspicuously competed in their contributions to this temple of the fine and performing arts. Raphael and Rembrandt, Monet and Manet are all well represented. During the autumn and winter symphony season get reacquainted with Bach, Mozart, and Beethoven. In the spring, dance takes the stage. Continuing around the PFA Circle is Vermillion College. Be sure to check the schedule for their popular Blackbox and Broadway theater series. The Academy of Sciences comes next with special exhibits on the wonders of the natural world. Hamilton Baptist University, completing the circle, is well-known for its choral music program and the extensive collection of the Institute for Near Eastern Archeology (3100 North Juniper).

The Palace of Fine Arts is on the northwest corner of the **Boulevards**, one of the most popular areas of San Luis Rey for both tourists and residents alike. In the 1920s more than twenty square miles of the urban core was designed, in the words of the architect, "to capture the spirit of early New England villages." Sixteen town squares, regularly spaced across a tree-lined grid, feature churches, schools, and all the shops needed to supply a comfortable home. A mix of town houses, bungalows, and apartments were designed to reflect the simple lines of timber and masonry homes of early America.

If you are not fortunate enough to live in these neighborhoods, you can get a taste of the lifestyle at The Boulevards Shopping Center. From PFA Circle walk along Juniper Boulevard, through what is justly known as Restaurant Row, six blocks to Buchanan Street. Don't be surprised if you can't immediately find the shopping center, but it is there.

The parking lots are tree covered. More than 100 retail outlets, mostly

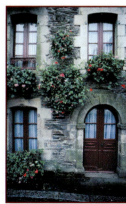

The Boulevards Shopping Center

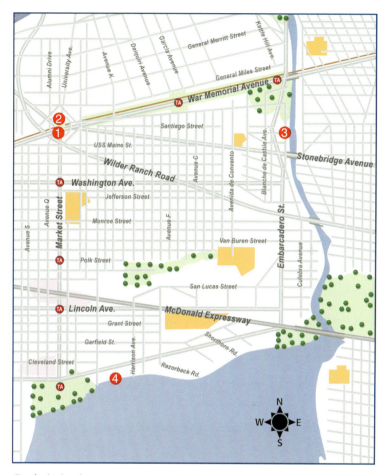

Top destinations in Mission-Uptown-Downtown include:

❶ *Soldiers & Sailors Circle*
❷ *Union Station*
❸ *Mercado de Embarcadero*
❹ *U.S.S. St. Louis Esplanade Pavilion*

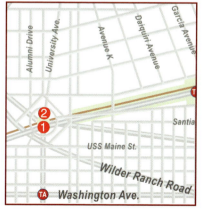

APPENDIX — SAN LUIS REY

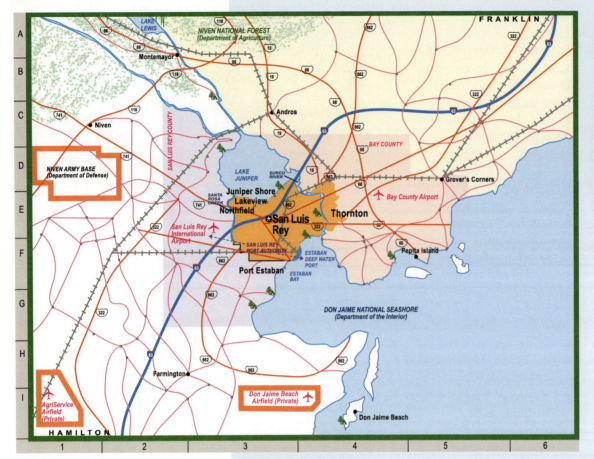

2,000 square mile view of the San Luis Rey area.

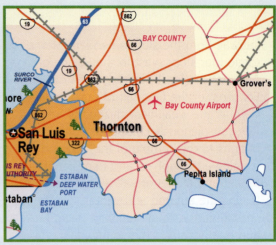

The City of Thornton is San Luis Rey's closest major metropolitan neighbor.

SAN LUIS REY FACTS IN BRIEF

Population:
- City 680,000
- Region 2,120,000

Area:
- City .... 280 square miles
- Region .... 2,110 square miles

Altitude:
- City .... 0–64 ft. above sea level
- Region .... 0–2,180 ft. above sea level

Climate:
- Average temperature .... Jan. 54°F, July 84°F
- Average rainfall .... 45 inches

Founded:
- City 1706
- Incorporated as a city 1846
- State of Franklin joins union 1843
- State of Hamilton joins union 1846

locally owned boutiques, are cozily blended into a lively residential community. Antique stores offer everything from 18th century French furniture to funky fifties castaways. Cafes, galleries, and working studios for glass blowing, jewelry making, and garden sculpture offer a unique range of shopping possibilities. Many of the boutique owners still live "above the shop" in this intimate village in the midst of one of the nation's largest cities.

These are only four of the dozens of "small towns" and unique neighborhoods that make up San Luis Rey.

SAN LUIS REY ECONOMIC PROFILE

San Luis Rey is a world leader in several **industries and services** including petroleum production and refining, insurance, banking, electric power distribution, biochemical research and production, health care, higher education, telecommunications, and shipping.

The San Luis Rey Metropolitan Region (population: 2,120,000) is among the 25 largest in the nation with an average household income ($50,800) nearly 15 percent above the national average. Tourism attracts more than 2 million visitors a year to the city.

The **Estaban Deep Water Port** is one of the top ten in the United States in terms of dollar value of imports and exports, and features a unique free trade zone that could substantially reduce your costs and increase your profits. This is the only major port in the continental United States featuring "greenfield development" over the last decade. No other American port exceeds Estaban's intermodal efficiency.

In 2000 the Board of Education of San Luis Rey was recognized by the Evelyn Proctor Foundation for excellence in urban **education**. A higher percentage of eighteen-year-olds complete a high school diploma than in any other of the fifty largest metropolitan regions of the United States. San Luis Rey is home to four universities and colleges enrolling over 40,000 students. The San Luis Rey State University Graduate School of Business has been recognized by *Excel Magazine* as one of the top schools in the region for financial management and strategic planning.

For nearly a century the **Lake Juniper Water Authority** (LJWA) has led a strong public-private partnership in producing clean and abundant electricity for the region. LJWA has some of the lowest rates and strongest service records of any electric power utility in the United States.

When Hester Pharmaceuticals needed access to clean water, it chose urban San Luis Rey for a new state-of-the-art production facility. The Santa Rosa Spring produces a natural mineral water savored around the world.

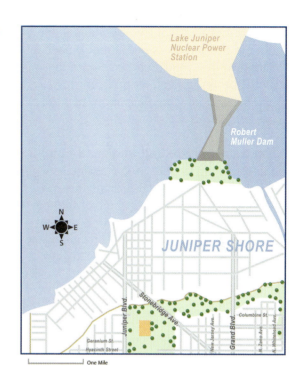

Locally founded NGTT Corporation is one of the top five providers of Internet broadband access in the world. San Luis Rey is the global center for its fiber optic, microwave, and satellite network. Talk about point of presence!

San Luis Rey is the **rail and road hub** for the states of Hamilton and Franklin, serving a population of over 18 million. The Port Authority Truck Terminal is among the top ten in the nation in terms of volume. San Luis Rey International Airport provides daily non-stop connections to Atlanta, Newark, Chicago, Los Angeles, San Francisco, Mexico City, and Amsterdam.

SAN LUIS REY HISTORY

Father Hidalgo Estaban arrived near the site of present day San Luis Rey on August 25, 1706, the feast day of Saint Louis, King of France, for whom he named the area.

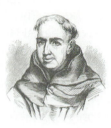
Father Hidalgo Estaban

In 1732 silver deposits were found in the San Gabriel Mountains. During the brief silver boom a small town grew up around the mission. By 1740 the Pueblo de San Luis Rey counted 1876 inhabitants.

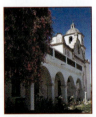
Cathedral of St. Jerome

The Cathedral of Saint Jerome was constructed in 1742-1758 as the seat of the huge Diocese of San Luis Rey. The Perichole Theater was also built during this period. The original stone bridge crossing the Surco River was built in 1754. There have been three bridges subsequently built on the same location, the most recent in 1975.

In 1815 the region was annexed by the United States. For ten years San Luis Rey was the capital of the Franklin Territory. In 1846 the State of Hamilton joined the union, but the capital was moved to Alexander City.

Following the Civil War the region saw a significant increase in population, mostly from the former Confederate States of America. By 1870 the population of San Luis Rey had increased to 27,000. The production and processing of cotton brought new wealth to the region in the late 19th Century.

By 1875 the Cotton Exchange, then located on the Avenida de Convento, had become the largest spot market for cotton in the world. The new cotton barons began building elaborate homes along the bluffs above the river bottom city. In 1890 a devastating flood destroyed most of the homes and businesses south of Presidio Avenue, and a new commercial district emerged on the bluff at the head of an extended Stonebridge Avenue.

In 1890 South County rancher Thornton Wilder discovered oil on his property. Wilder and oil together would transform the San Luis Rey region.

By 1895 the Wilder Ranch Field was producing more oil than any other oil field in the United States. Wilder and other cattle ranchers and cotton farmers were suddenly very wealthy. In 1893 Wilder and his family, including his 18-year-old son, Thaddeus, attended the World Columbian Exhibition in Chicago. Inspired by the world fair, Thaddeus went on to study architecture at Harvard, where in 1898 he joined the

APPENDIX — SAN LUIS REY

Rough Riders and was killed during the attack at Kettle Hill.

As a memorial to his slain son, Thornton Wilder donated 1200 acres of ranch land to the City of San Luis Rey with the understanding that it would be developed as a new civic center, featuring a Soldiers and Sailors Memorial to those who died in the Spanish American War.

The donation also required the adoption of a master plan and architectural standards for construction. The result is one of the most architecturally coherent center cities in the nation, and a treasure house of early 20th Century urban architecture.

In 1908 the construction of the **Robert Muller Dam** formed Lake Juniper. This reduced the threat of flooding, produced an assured source of water for the growing metropolitan area, and was a source of hydroelectric power. A second hydroelectric dam was built ten miles above Lake Juniper in 1938.

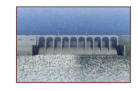

Oil production, petroleum refining, agriculture, and trade produced a sustained economic boom for the San Luis Rey region from the 1890s to well into the 1920s. A mid1920s effort to integrate the county and city of San Luis Rey only partially succeeded. Six suburbs (the West Towns) voted to join the City. But four other towns rejected the measure. The 1926 annexation of the former suburbs nonetheless created one of the largest municipal jurisdictions in the United States. In the 1930 census the population of San Luis Rey reached its historic high of 726,000.

San Luis Rey State University, incorporating the former Hamilton Institute of Mining and Agriculture, was established in 1946. The undergraduate and graduate science programs were relocated to a new Cottonland Campus in 1964.

A renewed oil boom in the 1970s prompted the redevelopment of the Uptown District and the commercialization of what is now known as the University Park District.

The 1989 construction of the **Estaban Deep Water Port** resulted in a sharp increase in the use of the port, with increasing economic benefits to the region. Displacement of shipping and trading firms from the largely derelict Southbridge warehouse district to the new port, resulted in that area becoming a popular venue for artists and musicians.

The population of San Luis Rey increased by 5 percent between 1990 and 2000, the first increase in nearly 70 years. Much of the increase was due to recent immigrants from Latin America, South Asia, and the Middle East.

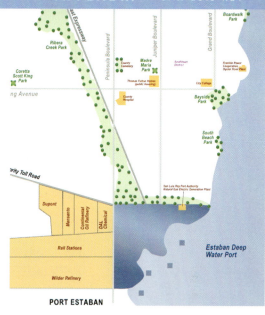

The Estaban Deep Water Port handles about 57 million tons of cargo a year.

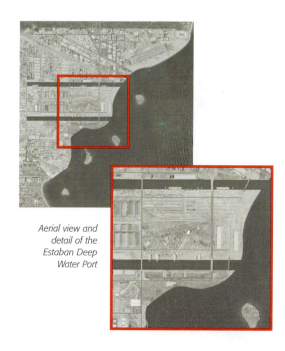

Aerial view and detail of the Estaban Deep Water Port

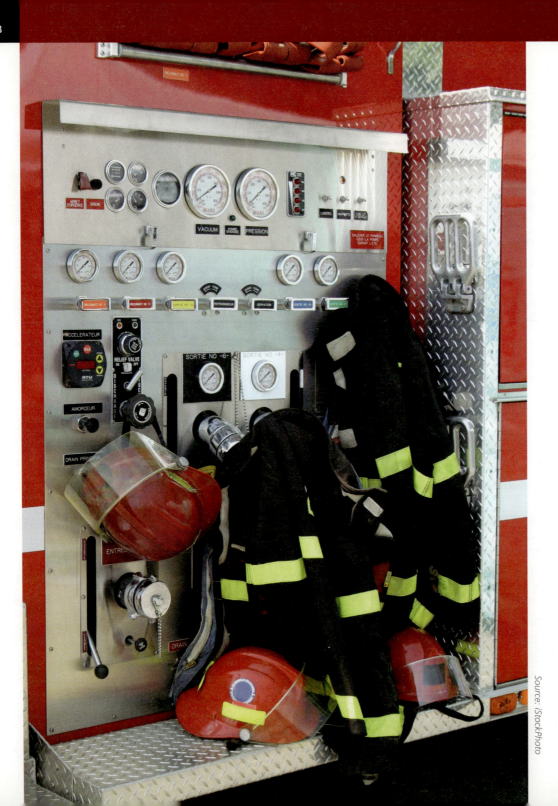

"The risk faced by firefighters warrants a concerted effort toward prevention of the terrorist act, rather than simply defaulting to response because 'that's the way we always did it.'"

— *Captain John Flynn*
New York City Fire Department

SUGGESTIONS

WE WELCOME YOUR SUGGESTIONS.

Please complete and fax this page to: 563-589-1819

Or you can send an Email to: homelandsecurity@mcgraw-hill.com

Your Name: _____

Your Organization: _____

Your Phone Number: _____

Your Email: _____

Your Address: _____
_____

In the next edition of *Catastrophe Preparation and Prevention* please make the following improvements:

_____
_____
_____
_____
_____
_____

I need follow-on resources for the Workbook:

___ An Instructor's Guide to include:
_____
_____

___ Sample Syllabi

___ Instructor PowerPoints to include:
_____
_____

___ Standardized Testing Instruments

___ An Online Discussion Board

___ Classroom or Station Posters

___ An Online Tutorial

___ Other, please specify _____
_____

___ Other, please specify _____
_____

___ Other, please specify _____
_____

___ Call me about some writing ideas of my own.

GENERAL INDEX

> **COLLABORATE**, **SHARE INFORMATION**, **RECOGNIZE THREATS**, **MANAGE RISK**, and **DECIDE TO INTERVENE** are referenced throughout the workbook. Please see the chapter dedicated to each of these principles.
>
> This index does not encompass resources available on the CD-ROM.

Apex fire, *54-55*
Avian Flu, *142*

Building Codes, *2*
Building Inventory Program, *2*

Capability Based Assessment, *29, 52, 55*
CARVER+Shock method, *40-41, 44*
Catastrophe, defined, *10-11*
Coleman Collaboration Equation, *96-97*
Community Emergency Response Team (CERT), *2, 95*
Consequences, *45*
Continuity of Operations (COOP) Plan, *135*
Counterterrorism, *57*

Delphi method, *115-116*
Department of Homeland Security (DHS)
    risk model, *38-39*
        investment justification, *147-148*
        vulnerability worksheet, *42*
Deter, *132, 135*

Emergency Planning and Community Right-to-Know Act (EPCRA), *53-54*
Exotic NewCastle Disease (END), *93*

Fear, as Threat Amplifier, *47*
Firefighter "Right to Know", *53*
First Preventers, *14, 17*
Force Multipliers, *53, 59*
Fusion Centers, *69-70*

Incident Command System (ICS), *93*
Intelligence
    Strategic, *52-53, 61-66, 127*
    Fire, *52*
Intelligence Process, *57*
Intelligence Targets, *59, 62-66*

Joint Terrorism Task Force (JTTF), *57, 61*

Likelihood, *35, 37*
Local Emergency Planning Committees (LEPCs), *53, 133*
London Fire Brigade, *13*

Material Safety Data Sheets (MSDSs), *134*
Mitigation, defined, *10*

National Strategy for Homeland Security, *4, 91*
National Incident Management System (NIMS), *4*
Natural, accidental, intentional threats, contrasted, *9, 17, 63-64*
Neighborhood Watch, *68-69*
Network, *65, 87-89*

Online Exercise, *22, 50, 83, 109, 130, 151*
Open Sources, *51, 77*

Positive Illusions, *20*
Pre-Incident" Inspection, *2, 54, 59*

Prevention Cube, *14-15, 132*
Preempt, *132, 136*
Protect, *132*

Risk, defined, *6, 36*
Risk assessment, *111-112. 116*
Risk Formula, *6, 35*
Resilience, *25*
Routine Activity Theory, *72-73. 101*

SARA, method, *114, 131*
Social Capital, *16*
Strategy, defined, *52, 57*

TALK method, *47*
TARA method, *124-125*
Terrorism, *25-32*, legal definition, *30*
Terrorists,
    Ideological, *26-27, 36-37*
    Religious, *26-27*
    Nationalist, *27*
    Issue Oriented, *27*
    Other, *30, 64-65*
Threat amplifiers, *25,47*

Urban Area Security Initiative (UASI), *38-39,103-104*
Urban Fire Storms, *106*

Vulnerability, *36*
Vulnerability Assessment Worksheet, *42*

Weapons of Catastrophe, *32-33*
Wildland/Urban Interface Working Team (WUIWT), *94*

Computer Requirements and Instructions for CD-ROM Companion to This Workbook

System Requirements

This CD has been tested for systems meeting the following requirements:

PC:
- Windows 2000/XP/VISTA
- Pentium II 233 MHz processor
- 64 MB RAM
- 800 x 600 pixel screen resolution
- Color monitor running "Thousands of Colors" or higher
- Audio capable system with speakers/headphones is recommended.
- 8x CD-ROM drive
- Mouse

Macintosh:
- Power Mac OS 10.3.9/10.4.8
- 500 MHz or faster recommended
- 128 MB RAM
- 800 x 600 pixel screen resolution
- Color monitor running "Thousands of Colors" or higher
- Audio capable system with speakers/headphones is recommended.
- 8x CD-ROM drive
- Mouse

Required Software
- Adobe Reader 7.0.8
- Adobe Flash Player 7

Starting the Program

Windows 2000/XP/VISTA

1. Turn on your computer.
2. Put the CD-ROM in the CD-ROM drive.
3. If the program does not launch automatically, double-click the Start_Here.exe file located on the root directory of the CD-ROM.

Macintosh Power Mac OS X 10.3.9/10.4.8

1. Turn on your computer.
2. Insert the CD-ROM in the CD-ROM drive.
3. Double-click the Start_Here file located at the root directory of the CD-ROM.

When you run the program for the first time, you will see the **License Agreement** for this product. You must agree to the terms of the license agreement in order to continue.

Performance & Troubleshooting

Ejecting the CD: The application runs off of your system's CD drive. Please do not eject the CD while using the application as it will generate unwanted error messages. Reinserting the CD will typically resolve the problem.

Technical Support
If you have any questions or experience any difficulties using this software program, please contact our technical support staff:
www.mhhe.com/support

Catastrophe Preparation and Prevention for Fire Service Professionals/Palin
ISBN 978-0-07-724077-6
MHID 0-07-724077-4

The 💿 CD-ROM companion to this workbook provides:

- Online exercises for additional learning
- Homeland Security resources
- Information about San Luis Rey®, the fictional setting for the workbook's scenarios

Details are below:

1. Online Exercises

Through the CD you can access the web-based "Homeland Security Terrorism Prevention Certificate for Fire Service Professionals."

This certificate is offered through the Institute for Preventive Strategies (IPS ©2006) at The Center for Rural Development in Somerset, Kentucky. The Institute for Preventive Strategies provides independent research, consultation, education, and training on the use of preventive-based strategies to avoid, mitigate and solve real problems.

The certificate courses are decision-based, scenario driven exercises that require the application of principles supplied in this workbook to complete. If you are a United State citizen you may apply for enrollment.

2. Homeland Security Resources

The CD provides access to the resources that are referred to in the workbook. In many cases, the full text is on the CD.

On the CD, you can use the "Chapter-by-Chapter" lists to locate resources that are referred to in each chapter, or you can use the "Complete References" list to browse all the resources.

3. Information about San Luis Rey®

Many scenarios in this workbook are set in San Luis Rey®, a fictional city that faces many realistic threats of catastrophe. The CD contains information to help you understand the city's risks.

San Luis Rey® is a registered service mark of Teleologic Learning LLC (www.teleologic.net).

▶ Passkey Code

You will need to input this passkey code into your online application for enrollment to the Online Exercises from the Institute for Preventive Strategies.
Your passkey code for accessing the Online Exercises and resources from the Institute for Preventive Strategies is:

MHFS-UFU4-GXCB-HHQS-UB3L

If you have any questions or experience any difficulties using this software program, please contact our technical support staff: **www.mhhe.com/support**